CW01394972

THE

NON-TINFOIL

GUIDE TO

EMFs

How to Fix Our
Stupid Use of Technology

NICOLAS PINEAULT

Interior Design, Illustrations & Photographs by Geneviève Gauvin, Co-CEO N&G Média inc.

Special Thanks: Dr. Martin Pall, Dr. Magda Havas, Dr. Anthony G. Beck, Brian Hoyer, Michael Schwaebe, Lloyd Burrell, Drs. Elizabeth and Marcus Plourde, Dr. Jan-Rutger Schrader, Dr. Martin Blank (R.I.P.), Daniel and Ryan DeBaun, The EMF Warriors, Dr. Joseph Mercola, The Environmental Health Trust and Carol Hiltner.

10 9 8 7 6 5 4 3 2

ISBN: 1976109124
ISBN-13: 978-1976109126

For a complete list of references and important edits that have been applied to this book since its initial release, visit nontinfoilemf.com/sources

For a complete list of EMF-related products I currently endorse, visit theemfguy.com

Mandatory Disclaimer

The claims made in this guide have not been evaluated by the United States Food and Drug Administration (and certainly not the FCC) and are not approved to diagnose, treat, cure or prevent disease.

This guide is not intended to provide diagnosis, treatment or medical advice. Products, services, information and other content provided in this guide, including information that may be provided in this guide directly or by linking to third-party websites are provided for informational purposes only. Please consult with a physician or other healthcare professionals regarding any medical or health related diagnosis or treatment options.

Inconvenient Disclaimer

Even though I'm legally bound to advise you to talk about the possible health effects of EMFs with your physician... the reality is that doing so will likely make them slap you with some kind of bipolar disorder and tell you to stop believing what you read on the Internet.

Most doctors have no idea that even very low levels of EMFs can cause side effects in some people — ranging from slightly affecting your sleep to the straight up debilitating symptoms experienced by people diagnosed with electro-hypersensitivity (EHS).

They took the oath of causing no harm... but they simply don't know what they don't know.

This EMF ignorance spreads way wider than just in medicine. Most home builders and electricians have no idea how to reduce the levels of EMFs in electrical systems they install. And most engineers and physicists still believe that low level EMFs cannot possibly cause harm — and have convinced most policy makers, politicians and influencers that anyone bringing up the issue must be a tinfoil-hatted, conspiracy-theory-loving lunatic.

Before our EMF safety standards finally catch up with what the latest independent science shows is actually safe, my real advice for you is to stay very critical, educate yourself, and do your best to reduce your exposure.

Affiliate Links Disclaimer

We've been practicing ethical, heart-based affiliate marketing for more than 5 years — and it's the way we've been able to put food on the table while we educate thousands of people every single day. If you visit some of the links in this guide and purchase recommended products, understand that we might receive a monetary compensation. We thank you in advance for your support.

Claim Your Free Bonus Report "5G In 5 Minutes"

Geez. Technology evolves so fast that I've written this book not even two years ago and it's already rusting.

Back in mid-2017 when I first published "The Non-Tinfoil Guide to EMFs", 5G — the 5th generation of cellular networks — was barely talked about.

As I'm writing this in late 2019, things have changed. "5G" has made it to the buzzword status and is now all over the news in many countries, and sparking a lot of concern.

Don't ask for a refund just yet.

I've written a short but very thorough report on 5G, which let's say acts as a bonus chapter for this book. Inside, you'll learn what 5G is all about, how it might affect your health, and what you can do about it — in only 5 minutes.

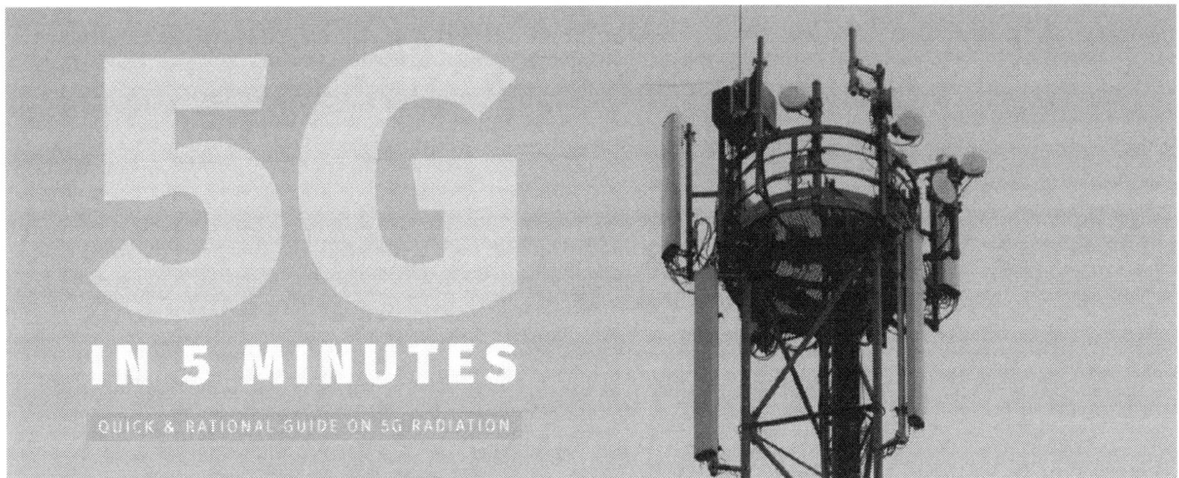

Simply visit the link below to claim your free bonus report:

http://nontinfoilemf.com/5gbonus

You'll also be subscribed to my newsletter where I post my latest podcasts, videos, and answer readers' questions. Hope you stick around!

Dedicated to the incredible human beings fighting to put safety before profits and to Maria August. I hope you finally found peace.

TABLE OF CONTENTS

Foreword

The Unexciting Story Behind This Guide

I wish there was an amazing hero's journey behind the creation of this guide. Maybe a riveting story about how I was holding my cell phone one sunny day, got so sick I was bedridden for months, and eventually discovered I suffered from a debilitating case of electro-hypersensitivity (often called "EHS").

Shortly thereafter, I would leave everything behind to become an internationally-acclaimed activist fighting for the victims of this crime against humanity.

The truth is... I'm just a guy trying to stay healthy, and who happens to be *slightly* obsessed with getting to the very bottom of things.

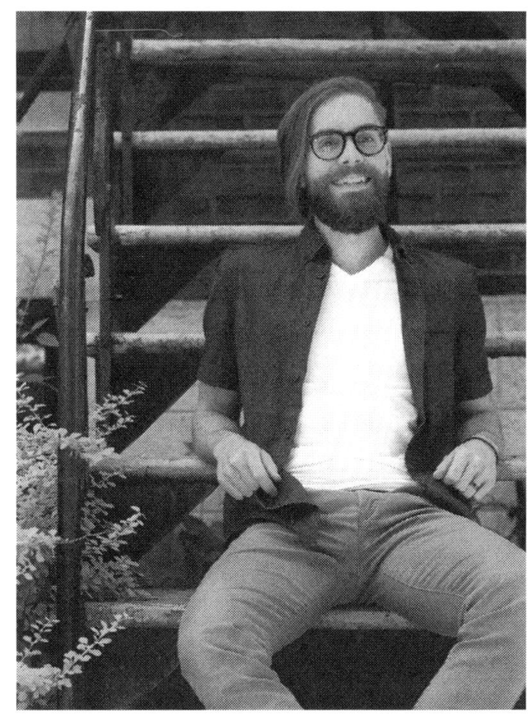

My name is Nick "The EMF Guy"[1] Pineault, and I'm a digital journalist-slash-copywriter-slash-online entrepreneur who has been publishing his findings about nutrition, our environment, and anything health-related on the Internet for nearly 10 years — if you count the year my mom was my only reader.

I've written well over 2,000 newsletters that have been sent to tens of thousands of people from all around the world. In 2013, I also authored an ebook series about our broken food supply titled "The Truth About Fat Burning Foods" — which has been sold in more than 50,000 digital copies. Based on these numbers, I guess that technically makes me pretty close to an Amazon bestseller.

Here I go trying to put forward my accomplishments in order to show you that I have some credibility. I hate it when I do that.

The truth is that I don't have special abilities or prestigious credentials — just a Bachelor's in communications, combined with an open, critical mind and the unique kind of stubbornness you

1 As I'm writing this in mid-2019, two years after my book came out, people have started calling me "The EMF Guy". You can follow my latest work on theemfguy.com

need to dive really deep in a subject, almost drown in the process, and eventually come back to the surface to explain the whole thing in a way that makes sense to the layperson.
This guide is the result of countless hours of research — probably well over 1,500 — studying the published work of amazing scientists, researchers, authors, activists and engineers who are studying the health effects of EMFs, second-guessing our current safety standards, and dedicating their entire lives trying to break up the status quo and make the world a better place.

My obsessive research process has included:

- Taking the best out of the top Amazon bestselling books on EMFs including *Zapped* (Ann Louise Gittleman), *Disconnect: The Truth About Cell Phone Radiation, What the Industry Has Done to Hide It, and How to Protect Your Family* (Devra Davis, PhD), *Overpowered: The Dangers of Electromagnetic Radiation (EMF) and What You Can Do about It* (Martin Blank, PhD), *EMF Freedom — Solutions for the 21st Century Pollution — 3rd Edition* (Elizabeth Plourde, PhD and Marcus Plourde, PhD), and *Going Somewhere: Truth about a Life in Science* (Andrew A. Marino, PhD) — just to name a few.

- Going through to the most recent work of pioneers in the world of EMF research like Martin Pall, Magda Havas, Martin Blank, Devra Davis (all PhDs), the Environmental Health Trust, Powerwatch UK, Microwave News, Daniel & Ryan DeBaun from Defender Shield, and much, much more

- Listening to dozens of interviews performed by Lloyd Burrell of ElectricSense.com with top researchers on electro-hypersensitivity, cell towers, smart meters, shielding, EMF mitigation and multiple other EMF-related topics

I would like to particularly single out *Radiation Nation: The Fallout of Modern Technology*, written by EMF pioneers Daniel & Ryan DeBaun as a reference for this book.

As I was beginning to write *The Non-Tinfoil Guide To EMFs*, *Radiation Nation* was released. Digging through this book sped up my writing and research process, because the authors have connected the dots in a way that had simply never been done before.

If you want to learn more about EMFs, all the resources cited above are very useful and will help you in your journey.

But if you prefer skipping the first 1,500 hours of research and get the gist of what EMFs are, why you should care, and what you should do to protect your health, then read on. This is what this guide is all about.

The Honest Truth About This Guide

The last thing I want is for you to read this guide and feel like you've wasted your time. So before we dive in, let's talk about expectations.

What this guide is:

- An actionable tool to help you learn what you can do today to safely reduce your exposure to EMFs and their known or potential related health risks
- An open-minded discussion about the overwhelming evidence which shows how outdated and ineffective our current safety standards are
- An easy reference you can come back to anytime, and that's written in a way you can actually understand
- Down to Earth education that's going to make you a healthier, happier person — whether you think you're personally sensitive to the effects of EMFs or not
- The definitive proof that we need to use our technology in a safer way while our standards catch up with the latest science

What this guide is NOT:

- An extensive, hard-to-read book which covers every single topic or health effect related to electromagnetic fields
- A political exposé on how telecom companies, regulatory agencies and other people are conspiring against your health (although there's definitely some truth to that)
- An engineer-level guide on EMFs focused on technical minutiae
- A book filled with out-of-context, cherry-picked activist propaganda and scare tactics about how you should shred your iPhone to pieces as soon as possible
- The definitive proof that EMFs are going to kill you, fry your brain, or give you cancer

Before We Move On

I won't lie — this entire EMF thing will feel overwhelming at first.

At one point, you might even get the intense feeling of an impending doom, and think the world is a very scary place — especially for those very sensitive to electromagnetic fields or small children.

But don't freak out just yet. Take a deep breath, smile, and simply do the best you can with the knowledge you have.

Armed with the new information you're going to get in the next pages, you'll be able to safely reduce your EMF exposure — 95% of which can be done for free, in just a few minutes. No tinfoil hat required.

Chapter 1

EMF 101

What's an E-M-F?

The 4 Types Of EMFs

EMFs Are Everywhere

What The Heck Is "E-M-F"?

When I asked a friend what's the first thing she thought of when she heard the letters "EMF", she told me she had no idea... but that it kind of sounded like "UFOs".

I quickly realized that even though the potential dangers of cell phone signals have been in the news for several years now — most people still consider that talking about the health effects of the invisible, odorless and silent signals we're exposed to from wifi, smartphones or any other kind of wireless device ranks pretty high on the conspiracy theorist, tinfoil hatted-scale.

To show you that EMFs have nothing to do with witchcraftery, let's go back to the basic science. And just as I tell my wife whenever she asks me anything health-related and is afraid my answer will turn into an hour-long monologue... "I'll keep it short. I promise."

EMF stands for "electromagnetic fields". An electromagnetic field is "a physical field produced by electrically charged objects".[2] Thanks, Wikipedia.

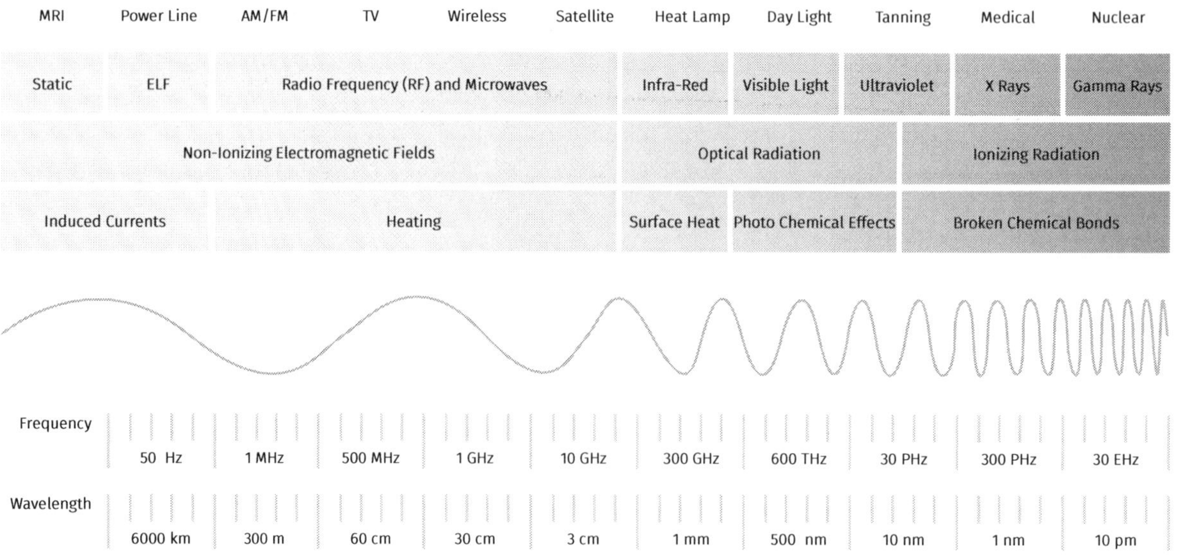

EMFs are organized on a spectrum, and classified according to their wavelength and frequency. On the left hand of the EMF spectrum, you find long waves with short frequencies like the EMFs created by a standard electrical outlet (60 Hertz in North America). On the opposite end, you find very short waves with a very high frequency like X-rays and gamma rays which contain enough

2 wikipedia.com

energy to destroy your DNA or pretty much instantly damage your body — and that you definitely don't want to mess with.

Here's a quick mind-bender for you: the frequency of an EMF signal equals how many times it oscillates every second — calculated in Hertz (Hz). While the Earth's natural magnetic field is known to be around 7.83 Hz, the 4G/LTE signal coming off your iPhone can oscillate up to 2.7 billion times per second (2.7 GHz). Now that's fast.

Now, we're still at the dinner-table conversation level here — because none of what I've said so far means that EMFs are dangerous per se.

After all, EMFs are basically *everywhere* in nature. Believe it or not, light is a kind of EMF, and the sun emits light in the visible spectrum (think of the entire rainbow), invisible UV light (helps you produce vitamin D or burns your skin if you get too much) and invisible infrared light (heat).

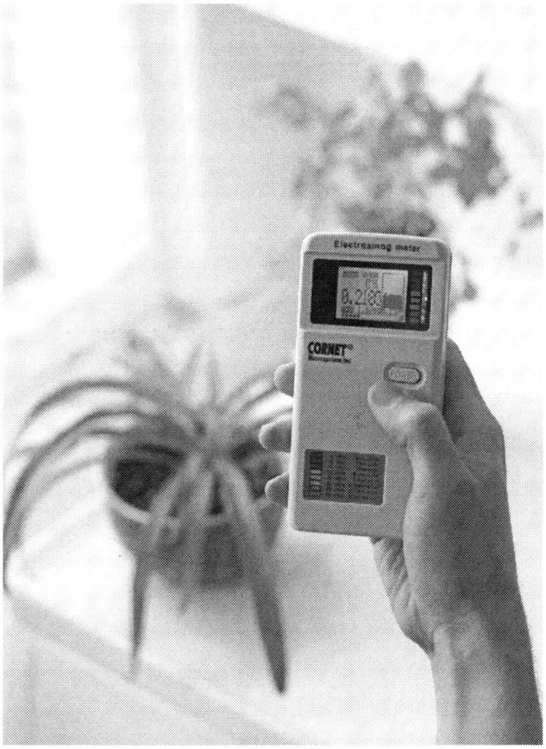

Part of the reason this whole topic is hard to grasp is that while a lot of animals are able to see infrared, UV and other EMFs that are invisible to the human eye,[3] most EMFs are invisible, odorless, and undetectable to humans except if you have a special meter like this very ugly but effective Cornet ED88T Electrosmog Meter I'll be using to give you real-life examples throughout the guide.

While I'll be talking about what we could call "natural EMFs" a bit throughout this guide, my focus here will be to look at the possible effects that man-made EMFs — generated from smartphones, wifi networks, cell towers, smart meters, everyday appliances, electronics and even basic electrical wiring inside your home — might have on your health.

3 sciencing.com

The 4 Types Of EMFs You Need To Worry About

I thought about calling these "The 4 Horsemen Of EMF Danger" or something fancier... but it just didn't sound right.

The first lesson here is that talking about "the dangers of EMFs" makes no sense — because it doesn't tell us *which* EMF we're talking about... gamma rays, x-rays, light, microwaves, or low level magnetic fields? The confusion is real.

Throughout this guide, I'll talk about the 4 specific types of EMFs that have been linked with adverse health effects[4] — Radio Frequency (RF), Magnetic Fields (MF), Electric Fields (EF) and Dirty Electricity (DE).

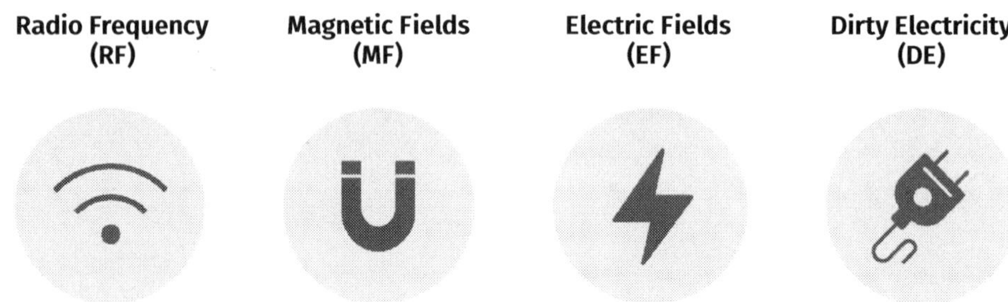

Look for these icons throughout the guide — they'll identify which type of EMF I'm talking about.

If you hired an EMF mitigation expert like a Certified Building Biologist[5] — these are the 4 main types of EMFs they would measure and try to reduce inside your house in order to make it a healthy, healing environment where you sleep like a baby and thrive.

Each of these 4 types of EMFs have been linked to specific health effects (both positive and negative), are emitted by specific sources, and can be reduced or avoided using specific strategies.

This might all be way over your head right now, but I promise it will start making more and more sense as you progress through the guide — so stick with me here!

4 Some would argue that this classification is way too vague, but I took the editorial decision to focus on the 4 types of EMFs most EMF mitigation experts and EMF consultants usually tend to address.

5 Building Biology is a profession which originates from Germany, and whose mission is to "help create healthy homes, schools, and workplaces, free of toxins in the indoor air and tap water, and electromagnetic pollutants." See hbelc.org/about for more details.

Radio Frequency (RF)

AM/FM	TV	Wireless	Satellite
Radiofrequency (RF) and Microwaves			

Common Sources of RF Radiation[6]

Cordless Phones	Smart Meters	Smart Phone (3G/4G/LTE)	Wifi	Microwave Oven	5G (next generation of networks)[7]	Bluetooth Devices
900 MHz	900 MHz to 2.4 GHz	710 MHz to 2.7 GHz	2.4 or 5.8 GHz	2.45 GHz	3.85 to 71 GHz	2.4 to 2.485 GHz

Ever come across the story a while back about how someone used a cell phone to cook an egg?

While it's an urban legend — the signal coming off your smartphone does't have enough power to prepare you a nice breakfast — there's actually some truth to that.

Cell phones, cordless phones, anything wifi, wireless "smart" utility meters and any kind of Bluetooth device all emit EMF radiation in the RF range — and some of them use the exact same frequency used by your microwave oven to cook food (although they use a much, much lower power).

The frequency of RF signals is fairly high compared to the other 3 types I'll talk about below — and range from 3 kHz to 300 GHz. Microwaves are a kind of RF signal ranging from 100 kHz to 300 GHz, so they're often lumped in the "RF" radiation category. Don't worry... none of this will be on the exam.

---

6 wpsantennas.com

7 At the time of this writing, it's still very unclear what exact frequencies will be used by 5G networks in the future.

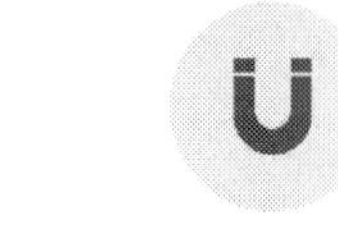

Magnetic Fields (MF)

MRI	Power Line
Static	ELF

Common Sources of Magnetic Fields (MF)

Charger For Electronics	High Voltage Power Line	Electrical Panel	House With Faulty Wiring	Electric Current On Water Or Gas Pipes

Any amount of electricity that runs in a wire or any other metallic object (like a water pipe, or a gas line — we'll address those later) creates an *electro-magnetic* field. As the name implies, this field contains both a magnetic field and an electric field that's perpendicular to it. It's science!

As Oram Miller, Certified Building Biology Environmental Consultant and Electromagnetic Radiation Specialist based in Los Angeles explains,[8] the most common sources of magnetic field exposure are from what he calls 'point sources' — including: "transformers, electric motors and your breaker panel and electric meters (whether it is a digital smart meter or an older analog mechanical meter). Point sources have high magnetic field exposure levels, but the good news is the field strength drops off rather quickly."

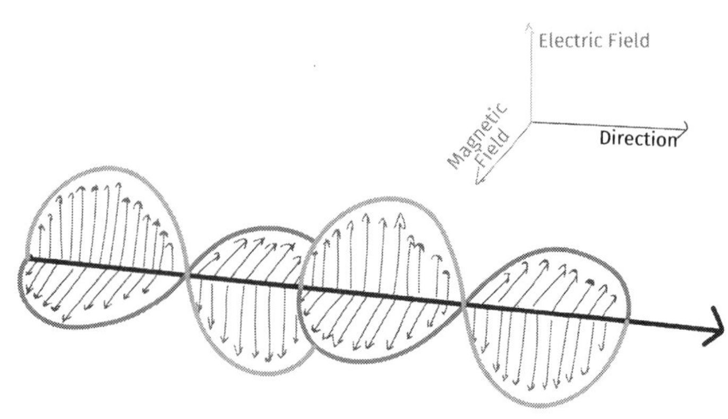

8 createhealthyhomes.com

What Oram means by “transformer” is obviously not “giant robot saving the planet”, but that any electronic or electric charger or motor which transforms the alternating current (AC) coming out of a standard 120/240v wall outlet into the direct current (DC) electronic devices need to properly run creates a magnetic field that can irradiate for up to several feet around it.

These transformers include the chargers you use for your smartphone and your laptop, just to name two.

The Magnetic Fields I'll focus on throughout this guide about are those in the 50-60 Hz range — mostly created by the electricity running through any appliance or electronic device inside your home and that can be a problem if you spend too much time getting exposed to high levels.

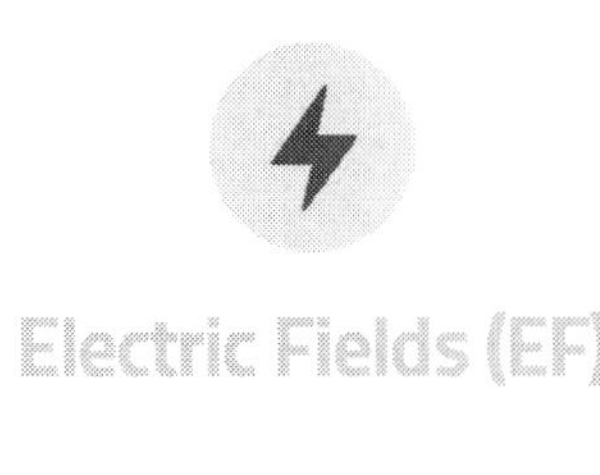

Electric Fields (EF)

MRI	Power Line
Static	ELF

Common Sources of Electic Fields (EF)

Household Wiring	Power Strips	Ungrounded Electronics	Cords & Chargers	Lamps & Lighting

To help you understand the difference between Magnetic Fields (MF) and Electric Fields (EF), imagine that you're watering your garden with a water hose.

How much water is currently flowing out of the hose corresponds to the current of the electrical wire — and creates a *magnetic* field around it.

Magnetic Fields

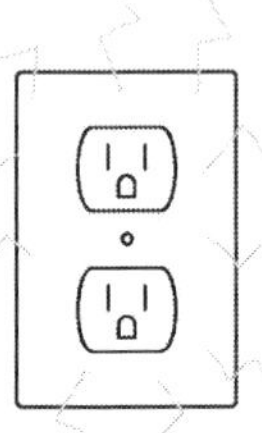

Electric Fields

The water pressure inside the hose corresponds to the voltage of the electrical wire, which creates an electric field all around it. Problems arise because this electric field is absorbed by the natural antenna that's your body — basically giving you a constant low-level electric shock that (in the long-run) can make you sick even if you don't feel it.[9]

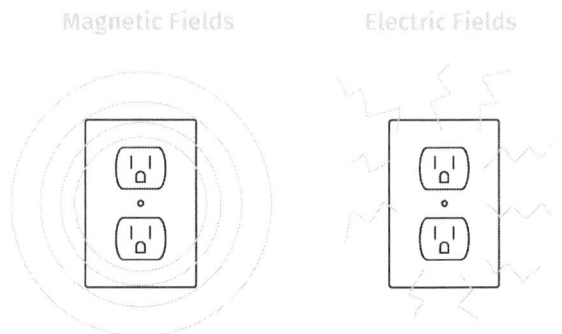

This means that just like the pressure inside a hose, the electricity inside the cord of a lamp that's not even turned "ON" constantly emits an electric field.

9 sparkburmaster.com

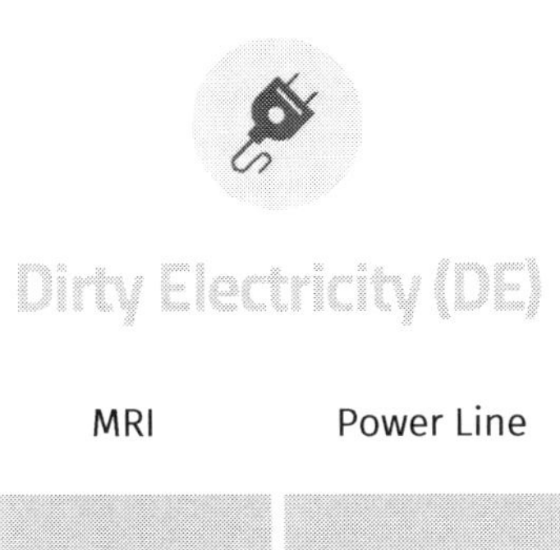

Static | ELF

Common Sources of Dirty Electricity (DE)

CFL Or Fluorescent Light Bulbs	Chargers For Electronics	Solar Panel Inverters	Dimmer Switches	Smart Televisions

Normally, the electricity inside the wires running through the walls of your home, workplace or anywhere else is supposed to oscillate at a frequency of 60 Hz (North America) or 50 Hz (Europe, most of Africa, most of Asia, most of South America and Australia[10]).

The problem is that a ton of modern electrical equipment has been specifically designed to operate by interrupting the current flow of electricity many times per second. A dimmer switch, for example, basically messes around with the ON and OFF button of your light bulb around 120 times per second. While your eye can't detect this very fast flicker, the end result is that this reduces the intensity of the light in your room.

Anything "energy efficient" works the exact same way. A compact fluorescent light bulb (CFL), for example, saves energy by going ON and OFF at least 20,000 times per second.[11]

While interrupting current this way can help us dim lights or save energy, this also corrupts the electricity, or as Dr. Sam Milham — an epidemiologist who has published dozens of research papers on the subject in the world's most prestigious journals for the last 50 years — puts it, "creates Dirty Electricity".

Instead of staying within the usual 50-60 Hz range, Dirty Electricity is a bum who likes to emit

10 en.wikipedia.org
11 Milham, S., MD. (2012). *Dirty Electricity: Electrification and the Diseases of Civilization*. iUniverse

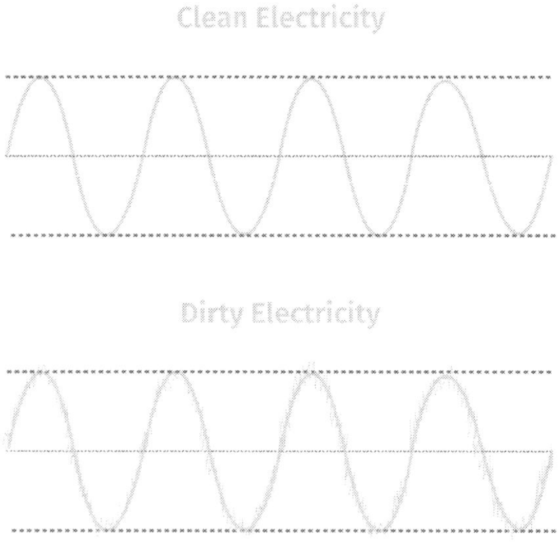

Clean Electricity

Dirty Electricity

a lot of EMFs in what are called the intermediate frequencies — ranging from 300 Hz to 10 MHz.[12]

What this all means in plain English: when the electricity in your home or workplace is dirty, it constantly irradiates these spikes of intermediate frequency Electric Fields which can have serious health effects according to Milham — especially those between 2 kHz and 100 kHz in the Radio Frequency (RF) range.

12 See Magda Havas' video "Dirty Electricity Explained" at youtube.com/watch?v=vbebpRvwd8k

We Live In A Big EMF Soup

Unless you decided to live off the grid, never use a smartphone, destroy your wifi router and stick to candlelight inside your home — you're constantly getting exposed to man-made EMFs, at levels millions of times higher than what you would naturally be exposed to in nature.

As I'm writing these lines, my cool-looking wireless mouse is emitting a 2.4 GHz RF signal at a pulse of 500 times a second[13] in order connect with my MacBook Pro laptop. This radiation is likely going all the way through my right hand.

Type of EMF	Natural EMF Levels[14]	Modern EMF Levels	Increase In Exposure
Radio Frequency (RF)	<0.00002 V/m	0.434[15] (background exposure in a city)	2,170,000%
Magnetic Fields (MF)	0.000002 mG	<2 mG[16] (average in US homes)	100,000,000%
Electric Fields (EF)	0.0001 V/m	<10 V/m[17] (average in US homes)	10,000,000%

My headphones are producing a weak magnetic field that reaches the outer layer of my brain. The Starbucks where I'm doing most of my writing nowadays has at least one powerful wifi router, and I estimate that there is a minimum of 30 different devices (smartphones, laptops, tablets, e-readers, etc.) connected to it — each of which emits a back-and-forth RF signal with the router in order to provide us coffee drinkers with some Internet goodness.

Next to my legs, there are dozens of power strips and my laptop charger — all of which emit Electric Fields just from being plugged into the wall, and Magnetic Fields whenever they are actively charging a device like my laptop.

I haven't measured the levels of Dirty Electricity in the room, but judging by the amount of CFL lightbulbs that are used — it's safe to say that they're pretty high — irradiating everyone in the room with a good dose of intermediate frequency-EMFs.

Feeling overwhelmed yet? Yeah, let's leave this place and get some air.

---

13 gaming.logitech.com
14 As reported by Michael Bevington in *Electromagnetic Sensitivity and Electromagnetic Hypersensitivity.* es-uk.info
15 ecfsapi.fcc.gov
16 1993 exposure numbers. niehs.nih.gov
17 1990 exposure numbers. books.google.ca

Just outside Starbucks, there are high voltage power lines emitting both magnetic and electric fields that are very strong when you stand right under them — but that also irradiate for at least 80-100 *meters* on each side.[18]

I have a hard time figuring out where the closest cell towers or antennas are, but as I'm in a fairly large city I'll probably find a handful of them within my line of sight if I pay close attention — and each one of these generates one or multiple focused beams of RF radiation.

Like I said... we're all bathing in a huge, invisible EMF soup. Notice I didn't say that this is an inherently bad or good thing — we're not there yet. The goal here is to make you aware of the fact that even if you can't see, taste or smell them... EMFs are all around you.

It's Increasing... Fast.

The entire world is getting connected. "In India, the world's second most populous country, government census data reveals that more citizens have cell phones (53.2%) than toilets (46.9%)" reveals Martin Blank in his book *Overpowered*.[19]

It's projected that from 2013 to 2020...

- *The number of tablet users worldwide will go up by 121%*[20]
- *The number of cell phone users will go up by 82%*[21]

We sure love our wireless devices. As EMF engineer Daniel DeBaun reports in *Radiation Nation*:[22] "In 2016, The Total Audience Report released by Nielsen showed the average American spent nine or more hours a day using electronic media. Given that the average human spends seven to nine hours sleeping each night, that means that we spend around two-thirds of our waking hours 'wired'." Yeah, this sounds about right.

Unsurprisingly, a lot more people are looking to join the EMF party. By 2020, an additional 3 to 5 billion people who never had access to the Internet will go online for the first time.[23]

---

18 emf.info

19 Blank, M., PhD. (2015). *Overpowered: The Dangers of Electromagnetic Radiation (EMF) and What You Can Do about It*. Seven Stories Press.

20 statista.com

21 statista.com

22 DeBaun, D. and DeBaun, R. (2017). *Radiation Nation: The Fallout of Modern Technology — Your Complete Guide to EMF Protection & Safety: The Proven Health Risks of Electromagnetic Radiation (EMF) & What to Do Protect Yourself & Family*. Icaro Publishing.

23 huffingtonpost.com

All this added wireless traffic requires more cell phone towers, more antennas on those towers, and more wifi routers. In the US alone, the database Antenna Search[24] identifies more than 1.9 million antennas or cell towers — a number that's predicted to explode in the next decade.[25]

But towers are costly and cumbersome, which is why a total of 8 large corporations like Facebook, Samsung and Google[26] are coming up with creative ways to beam the entire planet with a RF signal — with the philanthropic intention to provide every citizen of this good world with free Internet access.
But why just connect every human being to the Internet? Our new smart electronics need it too! Experts in the development of what's called the "Internet of Things" (IoT) predict that by 2020, there will be around 50 billion devices, people or sensors connected with each other.[27]

These include your Bluetooth dimmer switches and home appliances, but also wireless traffic lights, light bulbs, cars (GPS, satellite radio, etc.), FM-emitting posters[28] and yes! — even wireless sensors placed on trees to be able to monitor which one needs to be watered.[29] Why not?

The Scary Question.

I can safely say two things at this point:

1. We are exposed to a lot of EMF radiation from man-made sources — at levels some say are approximately 10 billion times higher than back in the 1960s[30]

2. These EMF radiation levels will likely be thousands if not millions of times higher in just a few decades — unless we decide there's a good reason to control them

With this gargantuan (yes, gargantuan) and incredibly fast increase in the amount EMFs we're all exposed to, it'll be a huge relief to hear that science has definitely *proven* that EMFs cause no harm, and that cell phone manufacturers and anyone creating any kind of device which emits these never-seen-before signals is required to follow stringent Governmental safety standards.

Because science shows these things are safe... right? ... Right?

---

24 antennasearch.com The website is only available from the US, unfortunately.
25 rcrwireless.com
26 stopglobalwifi.org
27 diamandis.com
28 washington.edu
29 agrisupportonline.com
30 Olga Sheean, olgasheean.com, page 5.

Chapter 2

SCIENCE

Why Scientists Rarely Agree

Good vs. Bad EMF Science

Am I A "Cherry Picker"?

Science Reality Check

I remember the day my two brothers and I found Christmas gifts in my parents' closet.

At that very moment, I was faced with a dilemma... either live in denial and continue to believe Santa is real, or face the reality that Santa doesn't actually exist, but that what really counts about Christmas is getting to see people you love and the genuine joy you feel when giving or receiving a gift.

This is pretty much what's going to happen in the next few seconds — because I'm here to tell you the guy called "Science" doesn't actually exist.

Even though I personally make that mistake more often than I'd like, saying stuff like "science says..." or "science has proven" makes no sense whatsoever.

Science is not a thing, or a person. If it were a real person, it would be the weirdest bipolar guy I've ever met — someone who's clearly unstable, unpredictable, probably dangerous and who seems to change his mind every other day.

Sounds familiar? One day, a study comes out that definitely proves that cell phones cause brain cancer. The next day, it seems that freaking tomatoes cause cancer too. Guess that means we'll eat dry spaghetti tonight...

Then, the next week, FOX News, CNN and a thousand media outlets start quoting a different expert from a different study who tells the world how "there's no link between cell phone use and cancer."[31] So... who's right?

Stop believing that science is black or white. It's not. Like all of us, it's a hot, imperfect mess — that hopefully does most things right, but that makes a ton of mistakes, wastes time doing the wrong things, says things it regrets, and is struck with inner conflict way more often than it'd like.

---

31 nhs.uk

Good EMF Science vs. Bad EMF Science

If you want to learn all about the history of how our current EMF safety standards came to be, how researchers, policy makers and scientists are imperfect, often biased human beings too, and how science isn't all about sparkles and unicorns — you have to read Andrew Marino's *Going Somewhere*. It's so eye-opening it almost hurts.

This guide isn't about politics, but talking about what science is and is not is essential to open your mind to the rest of the book — the fact that there's such a gap between what the latest EMF science shows, and the so-called "safety" standards protecting you, your children and the entire planet from their potential health effects.

If you feel like skipping this entire chapter, go ahead. But please don't send in hate mail (hello@nontinfoilemf.com) before you do so and understand where I'm coming from.

Still here? Good. To help you spot bad science from good science, simply ask yourself these 4 questions...

1) Are Researchers Really Independent?

When looking at all the studies demonstrating the health effects of EMFs (or lack thereof), we have to consider who's providing the funding.

As Martin Blank, PhD reports in *Overpowered*: "Since 1990, Lai has been tracking the studies of the health effects of RF radiation on humans published around the world. He has hundreds of such studies in his database. Approximately 30% of the studies are funded by the wireless industry and 70% are funded by other sources that are presumably more independent.

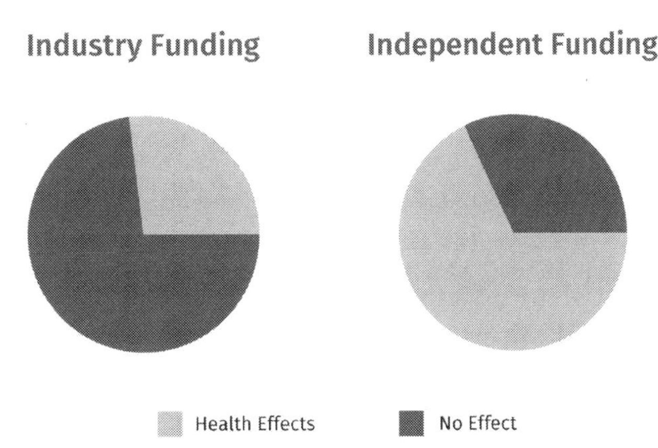

Of the industry-funded studies, 27% demonstrated a biological effect in humans resulting from RF exposure; whereas independently funded studies found such effects in 68% of the studies. As Lai explains, 'a lot of the studies that are done right now are done purely as PR tools for the industry'."

Now, this doesn't mean that all industry-funded studies are wrong, and that all independent studies are right — but it's an important observation nonetheless.

Another interesting observation is that a lot of different EMF researchers originally hired by the Telecom industry to prove that EMFs aren't harmful to the human body got "fired" (in other words... their funding disappeared nearly overnight) the second their studies showed the opposite.

Allan Frey

In the 60s, a biologist named Allan Frey working at General Electric's Advanced Electronics Center at Cornell University[32] clearly demonstrated that cell phone radiation can open up the blood-brain barrier (I'll get into what this means later).

As he explains in *Radiation Nation:*[33] "After my work appeared and others supported some of it, effectively everything in the US on these topics was shut down. Today you can't get funding to do anything of consequence."

George Carlo

Dr. George Carlo headed the $28.5 million research program funded by the cell phone industry from 1993 to 1999.[34] In 99', he started getting attacked and discredited by the same industry who had originally hired him. There's a lot more controversy around Carlo, and some of his critics argue he committed serious fraud,[35] but the fact is that these days he's trying to warn the world about the dangers of cell phones.

Om P. Gandhi

P. Gandhi is a researcher who worked with the industry to develop the "SAR" testing all cell phones need to go through before hitting the market.

---

32 cellphonetaskforce.org

33 DeBaun, D. and DeBaun, R. (2017). *Radiation Nation: The Fallout of Modern Technology — Your Complete Guide to EMF Protection & Safety: The Proven Health Risks of Electromagnetic Radiation (EMF) & What to Do Protect Yourself & Family*. Icaro Publishing.

34 emf-health.com

35 microwavenews.com

When he started talking about the fact that children could be at risk from cell phone radiation because their head is smaller than the one used during testing, he gently got informed that "if he did not discontinue his research on children his funding would be cut off".

Fortunately for humanity, he didn't choose the dark side and stuck to his values even if this meant a serious salary cut and a shorter and less prestigious career.

2) What Does A Study Actually Mean?

Mainstream media is famous for reporting studies with bold titles that simply make no sense — but that sure sell copies.

In 2016 — when the results of an Australian study looking at more than 34,000 brain cancer sufferers from the past 30 years, trying to see if there's a clear link between their cancer and cell phone use,[36] the media went wild...

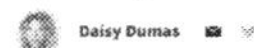
Mobile phone use not causing brain cancer, University of Sydney study claims
Daisy Dumas
Your Cell Phone Absolutely Will Not Give You Brain Cancer
No Brain Tumor, Cell Phone Link, Study Says; Expert Has Doubts
Roxanne Nelson, BSN, RN
May 12, 2016
30 years of data shows no link between mobile phones and brain cancer

The problem? As the authors of the study reveal in the conclusion... "The data the researchers had was about having a mobile phone contract – they didn't have individual patterns of use in terms of how often the phone was pressed up against users' heads emitting different strengths of radiation, for example. As such, it's probably wise to use the term phone ownership, rather than phone use – used in the media – when talking about this study."

In other words: this study found no link between *owning* a cell phone and dying of brain cancer — not that there's no link between cell phone use and brain cancer.

To me, the fact that researchers literally have no idea if any of the 34,000 brain cancer victims used in the study were ever exposed to cell phone radiation is pretty much sufficient to put it in the "useless study" garbage pile.

36 nhs.uk

I would personally put much more trust in the latest NTP study[37] which found serious increases in cancer on rats exposed to the amount of radiation you'd get from talking on a cell phone for just 30 days for 36 years — a much more realistic view of the issue.

3) Are people "Cherry Picking" or "Looking For Black Swans"?

Like I said — for every single study which links cell phones and cancer, someone could find a different study which shows there's no link.

Industry and governments would prefer EMFs to be safe, so each time a study which shows no link between EMFs and negative side effects, they wave it in the face of activists who are convinced of the opposite.

Then there's the EMF activists, me included, who happen to think that our current EMF exposure is probably unsafe. Each time we see a study which shows EMFs cause adverse health effects, we give each other a big high five, and feel like shouting "I KNEW IT!"

These are two classic examples of what's called the "confirmation bias" — or cherry picking evidence. When you're already convinced that something is true or untrue — you're always on the lookout for additional proof (and studies) which confirms how right and smart you are.

In order to avoid this mistake and spot *real* science from pseudoscience, famous science philosopher Karl Popper proposed that real science should be based on the principle of "falsifiability"[38] — always looking for evidence which might show that your theory is wrong.[39]

Let me give you an example. Let's say you take the hypothesis "All swans are white."

To prove this statement, most people would be tempted to start counting white swans. But as Magda Havas, PhD explains, "no number of white swans can prove the theory that all swans are white. The sighting of just one black swan disproves it."

A much better way to go would be to use falsification, and try to find a black swan. If you look real hard and aren't able to find a single black swan, you

---

37 microwavesnews.com
38 en.wikipedia.org
39 Based on Magda Havas' great video. youtube.com

can feel reasonably confident that your theory (all swans are white) is right — even if it hasn't been definitely proven just yet.

Now, let's apply this idea to EMF research. Havas continues: "How do we test the statement that EMFs are safe? We don't test it by counting studies that show no effect. This is the same as counting white swans, and is an example of cherry picking. Instead, we do it by documenting studies that find harm."

I'll refer back to this principle throughout the guide — because every single study which shows that EMFs do cause harm at levels well below our safety standards shatter the theory pushed by authorities that "EMFs are perfectly safe".

4) Who's Accountable?

Our entire society is built on accountability. If I steal something, the police will put me in prison or fine me. When there's a potential consequence to your actions or decisions, you generally think twice before doing anything stupid or harmful.

Following this logic, it would make sense that since regulatory agencies like the Federal Communications Commission (FCC) and the Telecom industry are both so convinced that the amount of EMF radiation we're all exposed to does *nothing* to the human body (which is totally false, or else I wouldn't have written a book about it), they should be accountable for the damage they could cause to every single human being on this planet if they turn out to be wrong... right?

Okay, this one is going to make your jaw drop. Since 1996, Telecom companies in the US are protected by what's called the "Telecommunications Act" (TCA) — which was obtained after the industry spent around $50 million in lobbying efforts.[40]

Two cool highlights from this bill:[41]

- Telecom companies cannot be held accountable if a cell phone antenna or tower ever causes negative health effects — AKA they have total immunity over health effects, and no one can prevent them from placing new antennas where they want.
- No one can tell Telecom companies to remove any kind of wireless service based on health issues if they stay compliant with the FCC guidelines.

40 As reported by Dr. Martin Blank in *Overpowered*. gq.com
41 repository.law.umich.edu

But What If?

I personally think it doesn't make sense to protect an entire industry from ever being sued over health effects — which gives corporations a grand total of zero percent of accountability over the safety of their products.

I guess it's somewhat pointless to debate this immunity, as long as the safety standards are safe — and based on good science.

I mean, imagine what would happen if our EMF safety standards happened to be insufficient, based on wrong assumptions or simply outdated... who then would be looking out for us and making sure bathing in our EMF soup is "safe"?

Chapter 3

ARE SAFETY STANDARDS SAFE?

How Your Cell phone Is Tested

7 Easy Ways To Stay Safe

Non-Ionizing vs. Ionizing Radiation

Meet Our "Safety" Standards

On August 1st, 1996, the Federal Communication Commission issued their FCC 96-326 policy titled "Guidelines for Evaluating the Environmental Effects of Radiofrequency Radiation".[42] That's the last time these safety standards have been updated.[43]

Remember 1996? I do. That's over 20 years ago, in a time I used to wear fluo shorts and when talking on this brand new Nokia 9000 wireless phone made you look pretty cool for a couple minutes — until you got exhausted from the sheer effort required to keep this 1-pound beast[44] (4 times the weight of an iPhone 7) near your head.

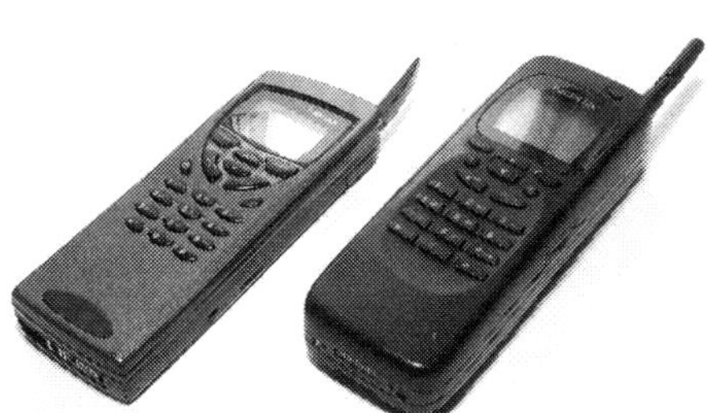

At that time, the FCC determined the following upper limits were "safe" for human health — mainly based on the recommendations of the Institute of Electrical and Electronics Engineers Standards Association (IEEE-SA), the International Commission on Non-Ionizing Radiation Protection (ICNIRP) and the American National Standards Institute (ANSI).

FCC 1996 Safety Guidelines For EMF Exposure

Radio Frequency	Magnetic Fields	Electric Fields	Dirty Electricity
1000 uW/cm2 or 61.4 V/m averaged over 30 minutes (in the cell phone/wifi range)	833 mG (milliGauss)[45]	614 V/m[46]	No known standards

42 transition.fcc.gov

43 The Environmental Health Trust points out that in reality, these standards date back from 1991. Go figure. See ehtrust.org/policy/fcc-safety-standards/

44 medium.com

45 The FCC doesn't have standards for the 50-60 Hz magnetic fields coming off electrical wires. The closest thing I could find are the guidelines from ICNIRP, which were 833 milliGauss before 2010, after which they increased to 2,000 milliGauss.
See pse.com/safety/ElectricSafety/Pages/Electromagnetic-Fields.aspx

46 The FCC doesn't have standards for the 50-60 Hz electric fields coming off electrical wires. Their 614 V/m standard applies to the 0.3-1.34 MHz range.

At the time these safety standards were set, a mere 16%[47] of US citizens had a cell phone, compared to a projected 82%[48] in 2017. The term "hotspot" meant, not a place with free and hopefully password-free Internet, but a place where two or more incoming RF fields cross and where you probably shouldn't hang out for too long.[49] Googling wasn't even a thing — Google was launched that same year. And no one was ever exposed to tablets, cell antennas or smart meters.

Let me suggest here that it makes sense to be concerned about the fact that *maybe* these guidelines were created for a world that literally had nothing to do with the EMF soup we live in today.

And this is not just my opinion. Hundreds of organizations, and even other governmental agencies (including the US Government Accountability Office,[50] the US Department of Interior[51] and the EPA[52]) have been saying for years that these standards make no sense.

Around the world, dozens of countries are following safety guidelines that are way stricter. China and Russia, for example, consider any RF exposure over 10 uW/cm2 or 0.614 V/m for 30 minutes to be dangerous[53] — 100 times lower than the current FCC guidelines.

But the problem runs deeper. Turns out that cell phone manufacturers can't even follow these already deprecated and loose safety guidelines. Let's see how this all works...

47 data.worldbank.org
48 statista.com
49 getvoip.com
50 gao.gov
51 nebula.wsimg.com
52 nebula.wsimg.com
53 who.int

Ever Read The Fine Print? I Don't.

What if I told you that somewhere deep in the fine print no one reads inside your smartphone... Apple, Samsung or Google is telling you *never* to hold the phone next to your head, or any part of your body?[54]

In other words, if you want to get exposed to what is considered a so-called safe amount of RF radiation coming off your cell phone (called "SAR")... you should never have a cell phone pressed against your ear, strapped to your arm, held in your hand, in your pocket, or in your bra.

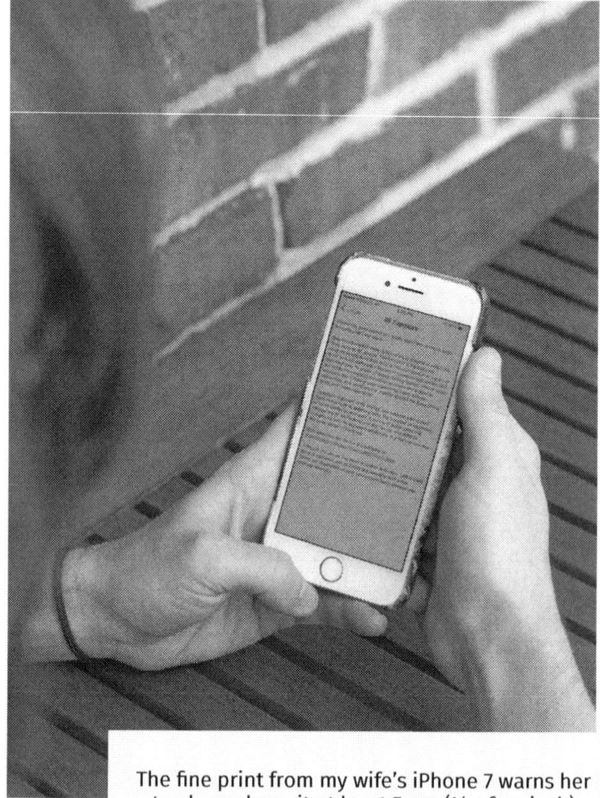

The fine print from my wife's iPhone 7 warns her to always keep it at least 5mm (1/5 of an inch) from her head or body.

What happens if you ignore this wise advice and hold your phone right next to your ear? As revealed by an investigative journalist who produced a great exposé broadcasted on CBC News' Marketplace, you get exposed to radiation levels up to 4 times higher than that phone's SAR rating.[55]

It's not very surprising, because RF exposure gets exponentially higher as you get closer to the source (in this case, the cell phone's antenna). According to world-class EMF engineer Daniel DeBaun, for each millimeter you get closer to a cell phone, your EMF exposure goes up by 10%.[56]

---

54 These warnings differ from phone to phone, and might have been removed or updated by the time you read this. See ehtrust.org/key-issues/cell-phoneswireless/fine-print-warnings/ for more examples of warnings used on different phones or wireless electronics.

55 Visit youtube.com/watch?v=Wm69ik_Qdb8&app=desktop to watch the entire show.

56 Daniel DeBaun. Interview with Tony Wrighton on the Zestology podcast, March 4 2017. See tonywrighton.com/never-carry-your-phone-in-your-pocket-with-daniel-debaun/

Any sane person would then ask... how can they get away with this? Aren't all cell phones required to be thoroughly tested for safety before being sold to you?

I won't answer this question directly. That would be too easy, and you probably wouldn't believe me. Instead, let me show you *exactly* how your smartphone is tested before hitting the market, and then you tell me how confident you are that someone is looking out for you.

Meet S.A.M.

Welcome to the RF Exposure Lab, in San Marcos, California — one of the many labs where cell phones are tested to make sure they follow the FCC guidelines.[57]

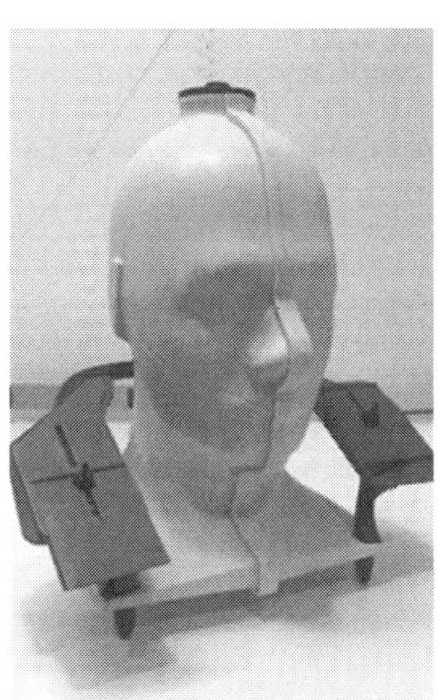

A mannequin head called SAM (specific anthropomorphic mannequin) will be our test subject today.

By blasting SAM with the maximum amount of EMF radiation that can ever come off your phone and measuring how much that radiation is heating his brain, we're going to figure out what's called the "SAR" rating (specific absorption rate — I'll get into this in just a second). Don't worry, SAM agreed to do this.

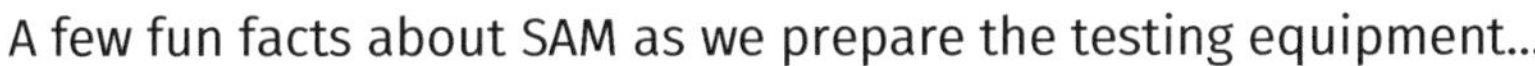

A few fun facts about SAM as we prepare the testing equipment...

- SAM is a big dude — the size of his head is based on the top 10% of U.S. military recruits back in 1989.[58] If he had a body, he would be 6'2" and weigh a solid 220 pounds — which means his head is bigger than the heads of 97% of all cell phone users.[59]

- SAM likes to hold his cell phone at least 5mm away from his ear, at a very specific 15 degrees angle. He isn't very talkative, and always spends less than 6 minutes a day on his cell phone.

---

57 rfexposurelab.com

58 electromagnetichealth.org

59 DeBaun, D. and DeBaun, R. (2017). *Radiation Nation: The Fallout of Modern Technology — Your Complete Guide to EMF Protection & Safety: The Proven Health Risks of Electromagnetic Radiation (EMF) & What to Do Protect Yourself & Family*. Icaro Publishing.

- SAM's head is filled with water. I mean, I would never even think of insulting this big fella — he just happens to have a head filled with a mix of water, salt and sugar which has been determined to emulate the average EMF absorption rate of a human brain.

- SAM also *never* uses a cell phone case. He just likes to keep things simple, you know.

Let's start the test! During 6 minutes (it's actually 6 or 30 minutes, but this is beyond the scope of our argument here), SAM's head will get exposed to an amount of RF radiation that's equivalent to the highest power setting your phone can ever produce.

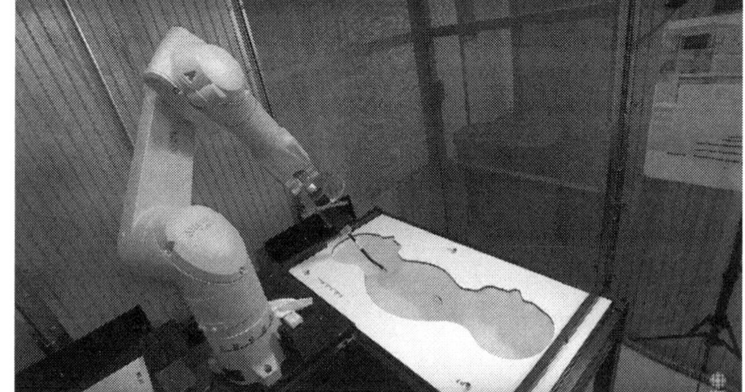

Then, a probe will look at how much the temperature in the middle of SAM's liquid brain increases.

If the measured increase of temperature is 1°C or less, we're all good — and the SAR will fall within the FCC's guidelines. This SAR rating is a measure of how much average radiation is being absorbed over 1 gram of human tissue — calculated in W/kg (Watts per kilogram of bodyweight).

But why 1°C? The original researcher who developed the SAR ratings, Om P. Gandhi of the University of Utah, observed that rats whose brain temperature increased eventually reached a point where they stopped eating. How much this is actually relevant to the effects EMFs might or might not have on human beings... I seriously can't tell.

7 Easy Ways To Stay Within The SAR Guidelines

Our test is completed, and luckily all the cell phones that have been tested fall within the safety guidelines, with a SAR rating of under 1.6 W/kg. Whew, what a day it was for science!

Before you leave, let's talk about the different ways to make sure you always stay within the SAR safety guidelines.

1) Be a 6'2", 220-pound military man.

Warning: If you happen to have a smaller head, if you're a shorter man, if you're a woman, if you're a child or teenager — you'll exceed the limits.

Children's bodies, for example, contain way more water than those of adults — which is why their heads tend to absorb up to 2 times more radiation from the same exposure compared to adults — and why their bone marrow absorbs up to 10 times more.[60]

2) Always use your phone at least 5mm away from your head.

Warning: Certain phones' SARs have been tested at a larger distance, so always make sure to look at the fine print inside your phone to find the right distance you should use. Also, always use your phone at the very precise 15 degree angle SAM uses.

Phone Model	Safe Distance To Stay Within The SAR
Apple iPhone 7	5mm (1/5")[61]
Samsung Galaxy S8	15mm (3/5")[62]
Sony M5	15mm (3/5")[63]
LG G6	10mm (2/5")[64]

60 ehtrust.org
61 rfsafe.com
62 rfsafe.com
63 support-downloads.sonymobile.com
64 10mm in the US, 5mm everywhere else. See lg.com/global/support/sar/sar

3) Only use your phone for 6 minutes a day, maximum.

Warning: If you use your phone at the maximum setting for more than 6 minutes, you'll exceed the SAR guidelines.

4) Never keep your phone in your pocket.

Warning: If you keep your phone in your pocket, strapped to your arm, in your hand, or in your bra — you'll get exposed to radiation that's not accounted for in the guidelines.

Also make sure you're never exposed to any amount of background radiation from any stranger's cell phone, any cellular antenna, any smart meter, any Bluetooth device, any wifi network, or any other device that emits any amount of RF radiation.

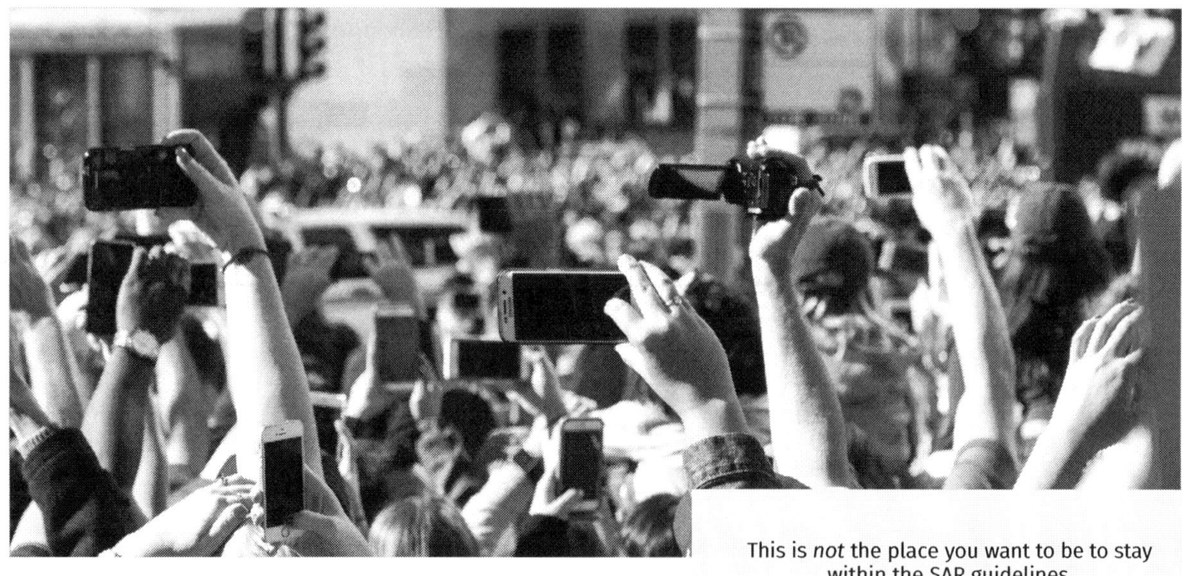

This is *not* the place you want to be to stay within the SAR guidelines.

5) Don't have ears.

Warning: The SAR is based on what amount of radiation gets inside your brain, and anything that gets on and in the ear on the side where you use your phone doesn't count towards the SAR calculation.

6) Have a liquid brain.

Warning: If you have a human brain instead of a liquid brain seasoned with sugar and salt, you'll pretty much automatically exceed the SAR.

After conducting the original SAR studies, P. Gandhi immediately followed up with a series of studies which concluded that using a homogeneous liquid to mimic the complexity of a human head isn't accurate — and doesn't take into account that certain areas like the bone marrow, salivary glands and the eyes are more likely to absorb EMF radiation.[65]

Maybe that's why the industry stopped funding him and even asked him to refund the funding he had previously received?[66] Who knows.

7) Never use a phone case.

Warning: As reported by the Environmental Working Group, using a phone case can increase the amount of radiation absorbed by your head by 20 to 70%.[67]

---

65 ieexplore.ieee.org

66 ethics.harvard.edu

67 ewg.org There are exceptions, and certain EMF-blocking phone cases are legit. Visit theemfguy.com to learn which ones.

S.A.R. = Still At Risk?

Clever title, I know. I smiled pretty good when I first came up with it.

In the last few pages, I think I've made the case pretty clear: the current EMF safety guidelines in the US (and Canada, and most other countries) are dusty, and no one on this planet follows them, ever.

Now, this entire safety fiasco is about to get worse — because it turns out that the SAR rating of a cell phone actually doesn't tell us anything about whether it's harmful or harmless to the human body. But let me explain before you burn this guide down to digital ashes.

As Martin Blank — a PhD who used to work at the Department of Physiology and Cellular Biophysics of Columbia University — puts it:

"The latest laboratory research indicates that the basis for the safety standards recommended by ICNIRP and IEEE is fundamentally flawed."[68]

What does Dr. Blank mean here? That looking at how much the radiation from your cell phone heats your brain or other tissues tells us *nothing* about whether it's safe or not.

In plain English...

The guidelines for RF safety are based on the assumption that any amount of "non-ionizing" EMF radiation that doesn't generate too much heat has no effect on the human body.

Why do people believe that? Because according to a lot of physicists and engineers, EMF radiation that's "non-ionizing" simply cannot physically affect your cells.

Have I lost you? I thought so. Back into the science class for a bit...

---

68 Blank, M., PhD. (2015). *Overpowered: The Dangers of Electromagnetic Radiation (EMF) and What You Can Do about It.* Seven Stories Press.

How Can Physicists & Engineers Be Wrong?

"Engineers should never be allowed to make statements about safety or disease in a human being."

- Prof. Trevor Marshall, engineer, published researcher and member of the Institute of Electrical and Electronics Engineers (IEEE)

Remember the EMF spectrum from last chapter? Since the shocking discovery of harmful yet invisible radiation by Marie Curie, her lovely husband and Antoine Henri Becquerel — for which they received the 1903 Nobel prize in Physics — scientists have divided the EMF spectrum in two distinct categories:

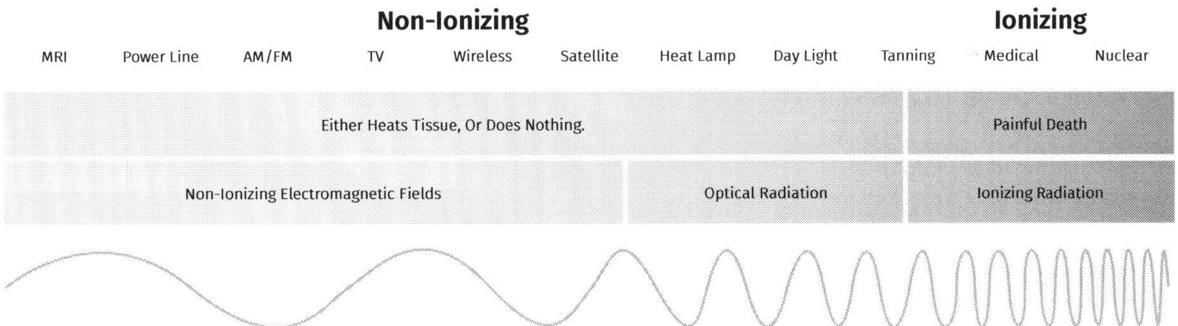

Ionizing Radiation: Radiation that "carries enough energy to free electrons from atoms or molecules, thereby ionizing them"[69] — which breaks chemical bonds. Exposure to ionizing radiation causes damage to living tissue, and can result in mutation, radiation sickness, cancer, and death.

Non-Ionizing Radiation: Non-ionizing radiation refers to any type of electromagnetic radiation that does not carry enough energy (photon energy) to ionize atoms or molecules. This radiation has sufficient energy only for excitation, the movement of an electron to a higher energy state.[70]

Now, the problem here is that while non-ionizing radiation cannot possibly break chemical bonds inside a human cell and instantly destroy your DNA — it doesn't mean that it has *no* biological effect, especially over time.

If physicists and engineers are so convinced that non-ionizing radiation has no effect whatsoever on the human body, it must be because there is simply no evidence this could be the case, right?

69 en.wikipedia.org
70 en.wikipedia.org

What's puzzling to me is that *thousands* of "black-swan" studies show the opposite — that non-ionizing radiation does have biological effects at levels way too low to cause any heat.

Let's hear from Martin Blank's wisdom again: "In 1948, two groups of researchers, working independently, both noted nonthermal effects resulting from EM radiation exposure. Scientists at the Mayo Clinic noted the incidence of cataracts in dogs following exposure to microwave radiation, and researchers at the University of Iowa noted that exposure to microwaves resulted in cataracts in rabbits and dogs, and 'testicular degradation' in rats."[71]

This is one of the thousands of studies showing that the 4 kinds of EMFs I told you about in Chapter 1 — Radio Frequency, Magnetic Fields, Electric Fields and Dirty Electricity — can either heal or harm even at very, very low levels.

We'll get into these effects very soon — but first let's shut down the whole ionizing vs. non-ionizing debate once and for all.

71 Martin Blank, PhD, citing the work of Dr. Zory Glaser. See magdahavas.com/pick-of-the-week-2-origins-of-1966-u-s-safety-standards-for-microwave-radiation/

The Debate Is Over: Non-Ionizing Radiation Induces Cancer In Rats.

If some skeptics and professional "debunkers" were still somehow able to argue that non-ionizing radiation does nothing to living beings — the study I'm about to tell you about has finally put an end to this massive delusion.

A $25M study performed by the US National Toxicology Program (NTP) studied the effects of exposing rats and mice to an amount of cell phone radiation equivalent to what a human would get by talking for 30 minutes a day, for 36 years.[72]

As reported by Microwave News: "The exposed rats were found to have higher rates of two types of cancers: glioma, a tumor of the glial cells in the brain, and malignant schwannoma of the heart, a very rare tumor. None of the unexposed control rats developed either type of tumor."

But here's the fun twist — because it's not the first time studies find possible links between cell phone exposure and cancer in rats... in the NTP study, researchers ruled out the heating effects by making sure the rats' body temperature never rose by more than 1°C. In other words, non-ionizing, non-heating EMFs have been shown to increase cancer risks in rats.

The irony is the whole reason John Bucher, the senior manager of the NTP study, wanted his agency to run this study is to prove once and for all that cell phones do *not* cause cancer.[73]

72 microwavesnews.com
73 microwavesnews.com

Freaking Out Yet?

I know I did at first when I realized the inconvenient truth — that there are simply no effective and truly science-based safety standards in place to protect you against the possible effects that EMFs can have on your health.

Now, this is the part where I could become alarmist and tell you to throw away your cell phone, because it can "kill you". Don't worry... it won't.

We know smoking can cause cancer, and still, millions of people still do it. Sugar is nothing good for my body — and still, I find myself being human and eating dessert once in awhile.

But the reason I don't stuff myself with sugar, alcohol or fast food is that it's now a fact that these things are not good for us — and that they need to be done in moderation.

So... how much EMF exposure is too much? How harmful is it? And what happens when we use the opposite of moderation and binge with this EMF soup 24/7? As Neil deGrasse Tyson would say: Follow me.

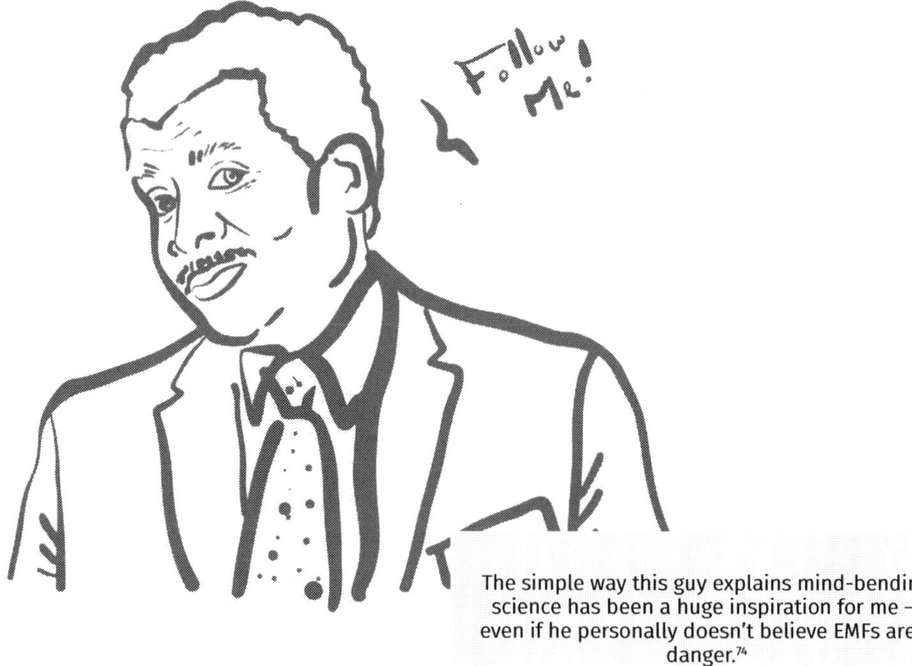

The simple way this guy explains mind-bending science has been a huge inspiration for me — even if he personally doesn't believe EMFs are a danger.[74]

74 youtube.com

Chapter 4

THE EVIDENCE

Your Body Runs On EMFs

4 Ways EMFs Disrupt Cells

EMFs & Your Sleep

Where's The Evidence?

If I flat out told you to stop putting a cell phone next to your head or anywhere near your body because they're harmful, your first question would probably be... "where's the evidence", "why?" or "says who?".

The main reason cell phones and other EMF-producing devices don't have a warning label similar to the one you can find on cigarettes yet is that the evidence linking EMFs to harmful health effects isn't as definitive as smoking and lung cancer.

Now, this does *not* mean there's no evidence. This means that from the hopefully very-objective point of view of regulatory agencies and the Telecom industry, the link between EMFs and adverse health effects isn't strong enough to justify having to spend trillions changing policies, safety regulations or how they do things.

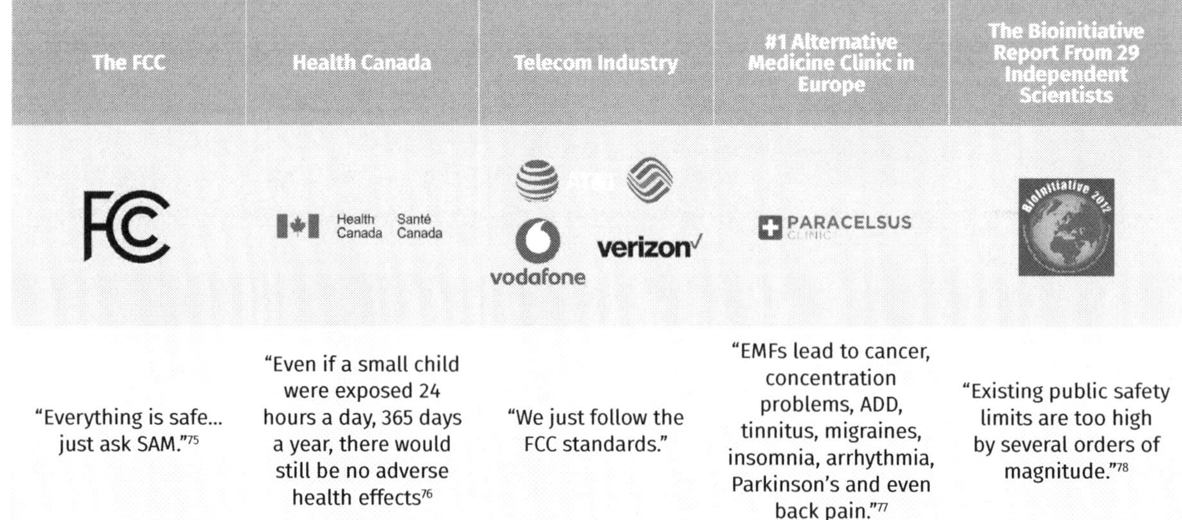

The FCC	Health Canada	Telecom Industry	#1 Alternative Medicine Clinic in Europe	The Bioinitiative Report From 29 Independent Scientists
FCC	Health Canada Santé Canada	verizon vodafone	PARACELSUS CLINIC	Bioinitiative 2012
"Everything is safe... just ask SAM."[75]	"Even if a small child were exposed 24 hours a day, 365 days a year, there would still be no adverse health effects[76]	"We just follow the FCC standards."	"EMFs lead to cancer, concentration problems, ADD, tinnitus, migraines, insomnia, arrhythmia, Parkinson's and even back pain."[77]	"Existing public safety limits are too high by several orders of magnitude."[78]

This is the perfect time to go back to the black swan example I told you about in Chapter 2. Remember?

---

75 Not an actual quote.
76 hc-sc.gc.ca
77 marioninstitute.org
78 bioinitiative.org

What the FCC and Health Canada are saying here is "all swans are white", or "EMFs cannot possibly cause harm at levels of current safety standards."

On the other hand, the 29 authors of the 2007 and 2012 Bioinitiative Report, doctors at the prestigious Paracelsus clinic in Switzerland and thousands of other scientists are saying "if all swans are white, how come there are literally thousands of black swans right over there?", or "how do you explain that a ton of studies *do* show health effects from EMFs at levels way lower than current safety standards?"

So while you follow me during the next two chapters — while we go hunting for these black swans[79] — keep in mind that our goal here is *not* to definitely prove that EMFs are harmful, but rather to disprove the assumption that they're definitely safe.

79 No swan, white or black, was harmed during the creation of this book.

Fact #1: EMFs Affect All Animals

"Any compound that causes chronic illnesses in animals should be regarded as if it could cause such diseases in humans."[80]

- The International Agency for Research on Cancer (IARC)

Throughout the entire animal kingdom, everything seems to be very sensitive to EMFs — both natural and man-made.

For example, birds can actually "see" the earth's natural magnetic field, which they use to migrate to precise locations at the other side of the planet.[81]

Insects are also very sensitive to EMFs, and display very bizarre behaviors when exposed to cell phone signals.

In a 2011 study, researchers also found that EMFs have a dramatic effect on the behavior of honey bees.[82]

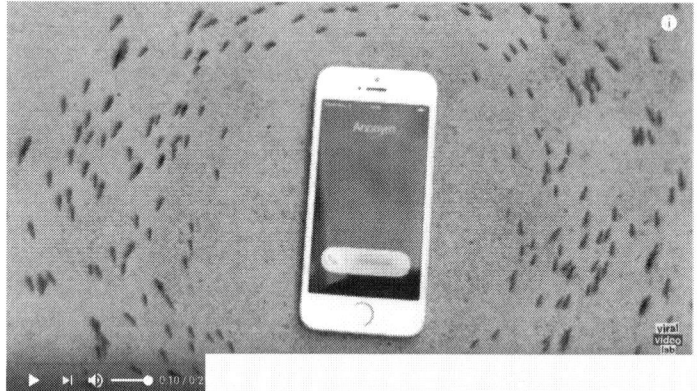

This video showing ants dancing in circles when this smartphone received a call went viral in 2015.

Some experts even think the increase in EMFs in our environment (think about the millions of new cellular antennas) is partially responsible for what's called the "colony collapse disorder" (CCD) — a phenomenon observed in the last 15 years where at least 50% of all bees have disappeared in dozens of countries around the world.[83]

When researchers from the Landau University in Germany put a cell phone near beehives, they observed that a large percentage of the bees never returned — probably because it interferes with

80 Davis, D., PhD. (2013). *Disconnect: The Truth About Cell Phone Radiation*. Environmental Health Trust.
81 nationalgeographic.com
82 springer.com
83 en.wikipedia.org

their navigation system based on magnetism.[84]

This could be the subject of 10 entire books, but the fact is that solid science is showing that EMFs affect every living thing on this entire planet in a major way:

- In a 2013 review of 113 studies on the ecological effects of EMF — 65% of the studies found EMF created alterations at both high as well as at low dosages. Of these, 50% revealed effects on animals, and 75% showed effects on plants — and the effects unsurprisingly got worse over longer duration or when utilizing stronger signals.[85]

- It's been known for decades that animals contain a natural mineral called "magnetite"[86] which can make them sensitive to 60 Hz magnetic fields that are 50 times weaker than earth's natural magnetic field[87], therefore 200X weaker than the 2,000 mG FCC safety standards. Birds have also been found to become disoriented by magnetic fields 2,000X weaker than FCC standards.

- Electricity expert Dave Stetzer has studied how high levels of Dirty Electricity in dairy farms can affect the health of cows in a major way. Along with other experts in electrical engineering and animal health, he concluded that "cows' behavior, health, and milk production were negatively responsive to harmonic distortions of step-potential voltage [AKA dirty electricity]."[88] He even found that reducing the levels of Dirty Electricity in a school 0.25 miles away from one dairy farm increased the production of milk by an average of ten pounds per cow per day.[89]

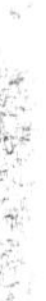

84 sciencagogo.com
85 As reported by Dr. Elizabeth Plourde in *EMF Freedom*. See pdfs.semanticscholar.org/7c23/70eabdb09a92a6663dec5e159e54cd84e86d.pdf
86 ncbi.nlm.nih.gov/pubmed/7213948
87 As reported by Dr. Martin Blank in *Overpowered*. See ncbi.nlm.nih.gov/pubmed/8074740
88 ncbi.nlm.nih.gov/pubmed/23416176
89 Milham, S., MD. (2012). *Dirty Electricity: Electrification and the Diseases of Civilization*. iUniverse

Fact #2: Your Entire Body Runs On Freaking Electricity

I guess some could argue that "common sense" is not a scientific argument, but judging by the fact that every single one of your organs relies on electricity and magnetism... it's kind of crazy to think that EMFs that don't cause your tissues to heat up do *nothing* to disrupt your health.

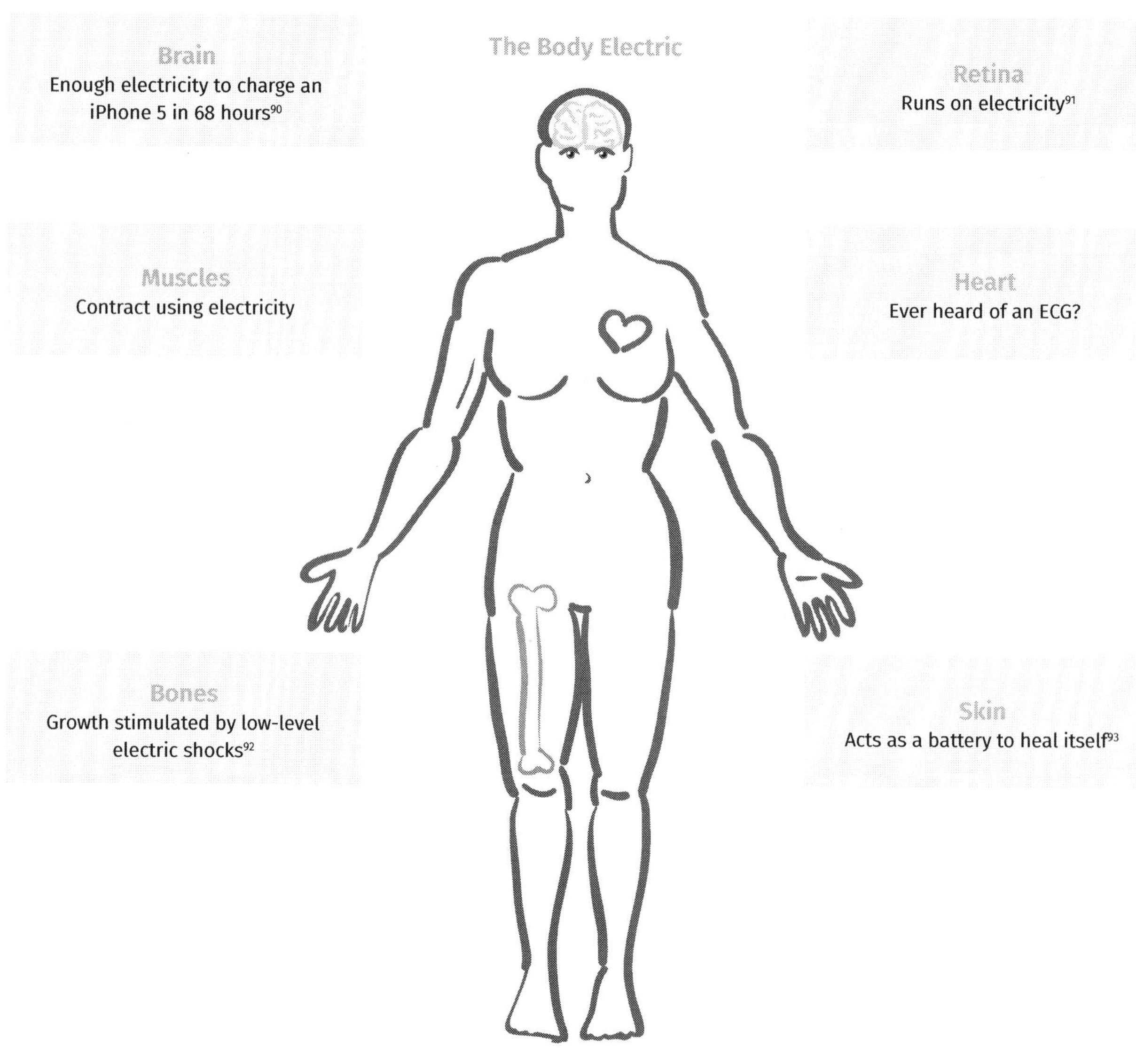

The Body Electric
Brain
Enough electricity to charge an iPhone 5 in 68 hours[90]
Retina
Runs on electricity[91]
Muscles
Contract using electricity
Heart
Ever heard of an ECG?
Bones
Growth stimulated by low-level electric shocks[92]
Skin
Acts as a battery to heal itself[93]

90 gizmodo.com
91 en.wikipedia.org
92 ncbi.nlm.nih.gov/pmc/articles/PMC2762251
93 onlinelibrary.wiley.com

Fact #3: Every Cell In Your Body Can "Feel" EMFs

The evidence is getting stronger. Not only does the human body run on electricity and magnetism... it turns out that every cell in your body has antennas to "sense" the electromagnetic environment around you.

In a presentation given at the Hebrew University Medical School in January 2017, researcher Rony Seger, MD, PhD explained that humans have the same kind of cryptochrome proteins, in every single one of their cells, that other animals use to detect magnetism.[94] This has been confirmed by many human experiments.[95]

While Seger is still trying to pinpoint exactly what part of the human cell acts as an antenna to "detect" EMFs, he has demonstrated that Magnetic Fields as low as 1.5 milligauss (1,333 times lower than the current FCC safety limit) and RF Fields as low as 4.34 V/m (14X lower than FCC) can activate specific pathways inside the human body.

For example, very low-level magnetic fields have been found to activate a pathway called "NADPH oxidase", which is considered a major cause of atherosclerosis, the hardening of the heart's arteries.[96] Does this mean EMFs can increase your risks of heart attacks? Be patient, we'll get into that in just a second.

94 Part of the lecture he gave at the Wireless Radiation And Human Health Expert Forum in Israel in January 2017.
See ehtrust.org/science/key-scientific-lectures/2017-expert-forum-wireless-radiation-human-health/

95 sciencemag.org

96 en.wikipedia.org

Fact #4: Every Cell In Your Body Gets "Slapped" By EMFs In Multiple Ways

"Nick... for all we know everything you've talked about so far means nothing. The fact that human cells can detect EMFs tells us nothing about whether it harms them. Maybe they just see the signal, shrug, and move on with their day."

You're right. Glad to see you're still following me here.

A lot of the mechanisms that could explain how EMFs affect different cells in your body are still very unclear — but four of them are very hard to deny:

1. EMFs Cause DNA Damage

"The belief that microwaves cannot cause bond breaking in chromosomes or DNA, or damage tissue more generally is quite inaccurate."

- Robert C. Kane, PhD, Former Motorola Senior Research Scientist

The reason there's no consensus about how EMFs disrupt human cells is that "Science" (remember... the lunatic from Chapter 2?) is still scratching its head about how our cells use low-level EMFs to communicate with one another.[97]

One thing is certain: our cells can sense the EMF soup we're bathing in, and probably go "Good morning, just another day performing key cellular functions — OH MY GOD WHY IS THIS PICTURE OF A CUTE KITTEN HURTING ME SO BAD?"

As Martin Blank explains in *Overpowered*, EMFs been shown to cause DNA damage over and over, "at levels of EMF exposure equivalent to those resulting from typical cell phone use".[98]

A 2005 study from the medical University of Vienna showed that a 1800 MHz signal (in the RF range) "induced DNA single- and double-strand breaks in both human fibroblasts and rat female reproductive cells. They reported that the intermittent, pulsing exposure showed a stronger effect than continuous exposure. In addition, they concluded that the DNA damage was not due to the effects from the heat generated."[99]

---

97 fluxology.net

98 Blank, M., PhD. (2015). *Overpowered: The Dangers of Electromagnetic Radiation (EMF) and What You Can Do about It*. Seven Stories Press.

99 As reported by Dr. Elizabeth Plourde in *EMF Freedom*. See ncbi.nlm.nih.gov/pubmed/1586990

This has been confirmed by research from Blank & Goodman in 2009,[100] and more than 10 other papers.[101] And according to researcher Adlkofer of the Verum Foundation, this effect is up to 10X stronger in 3G cell phones compared to the older 2G networks[102] — and we can conclude it's even worse in our 4G/LTE phones.

The most concerning part, explains Blank, "is that Lai and Singh found that the DNA in the rat brains continued to break down for hours after exposure ended.[103] This suggests that the exposure not only causes immediate damage, but also unleashes a chain of processes that continue to produce damage well after the exposure itself."

Now, it's true that a lot of stuff causes DNA damage — like sun exposure.[104] But while it's common sense to get the heck out of the sun before you get burned... are we ignoring our bodies begging us to get out of the EMF soup we live in 24/7?

Possible side effects from excessive DNA damage

Honestly, excessive DNA damage that's not properly repaired (and there's some evidence this could be the case[105]) could cause anything down the road — including cancer, premature aging, neurodegenerative diseases, reduced fertility, reduced immunity, heart disease or metabolic syndrome.[106]

2. EMFs Screw Up Your VGCCs

"What EMFs do in our bodies is that they work on some channels in the plasma membranes of our cells called voltage-gated calcium channels... What they do is that they open up those channels, calcium flows into the cell and it's the excess calcium in the cell that leads to all the biological effects that are produced by EMFs...

Autism is one of them. A second one is type 2 diabetes, the third one is the kind of cardiovascular disease that has to do with the electrical control of the heart... So all of the assessments of safety which have been based on the assumption that the only thing that these fields can do is heat things are based on a falsehood...

---

100 ncbi.nlm.nih.gov/pubmed/19268550
101 microwavesnews.com
102 Davis, D., PhD. (2013). *Disconnect: The Truth About Cell Phone Radiation*. Environmental Health Trust.
103 As reported by Dr. Martin Blank in *Overpowered*. See ncbi.nlm.nih.gov/pubmed/15121512
104 scientificamerican.com
105 ehtrust.org
106 ncbi.nlm.nih.gov/pmc/articles/PMC2906700/

Sorry, are my three minutes up?"

- Martin Pall, PhD, during a lecture given at the Portland Public Schools' Board of Education in 2013[107]

Another acronym? Really?

Yep. Science is all about acronyms! VGCCs stands for "voltage-gated calcium channels" — little doors that let calcium in and out our cells, and that happen to be powered with... you've guessed it... very low levels of electricity.

In the last years, Martin Pall, PhD from the Washington State University has extensively studied this mechanism and has published dozens of papers on the subject in the last 2 decades,[108] including a key study on VGCCs[109] that has been recognized as one of the top medical publications of 2013 by Global Medical Discovery.[110] In other words... the guy knows his stuff.

As he explains in a lengthy presentation he gave in Oslo in 2014 (yes, I sat through the whole thing twice),[111] very low levels of EMFs of different types (RF from cell phones and even magnetic/electric fields from standard electrical wiring) can keep your cells' VGCCs opened for hours after exposure — flooding them with extra calcium.

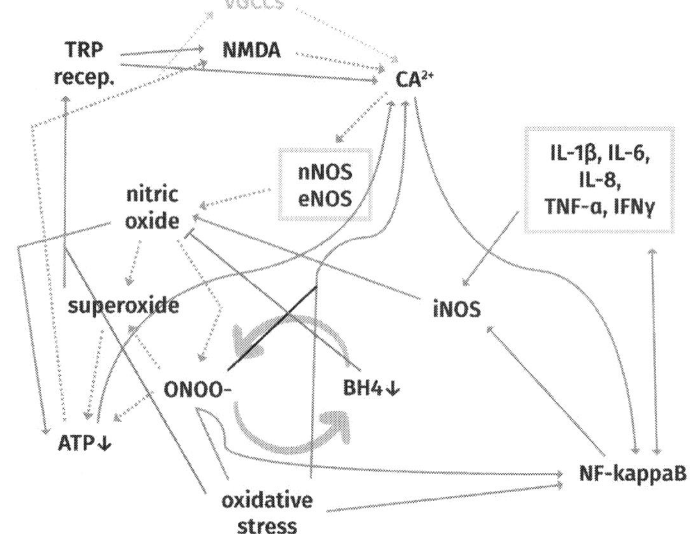

To understand what this excess of calcium can cause in your body, I'll leave you with this super easy-to-understand graphic Martin Pall came up with — which outlines the 5 different pathways that get disrupted and how they affect each other in synergy:

107 electrosmogprevention.org
108 researchgate.net
109 ncbi.nlm.nih.gov/pubmed/23802593
110 globalmedicaldiscovery.com
111 youtube.com

Just kidding, very few people (including myself) can understand any of this.

The important point here is that this excess calcium can cause a lot of downstream negative or *positive* effects in the human body — usually depending on which kind of cells in your body are being affected.

Effects Of Excessive Calcium In Cells	
Positive	**Negative**
• Bone regrowth[112] • Potential treatment for neurological conditions like migraines, strokes, Parkinson's disease, dystonia or tinnitus[113] • Potential treatment for psychiatric conditions like major depression or auditory hallucinations • As Pall explains, there are more than 7,000 papers show potential therapeutic uses for EMFs — all at levels too low to cause any heating effect (all positive "black swans"!)	• Development of skin cells[114] • Disrupts nerve cells communication[115] • Heart failure, arrhythmia, cardiac problems • Increase in cellular nitric oxide, which forms free radicals, oxidative stress and depletes the cells' antioxidants • Cancer • Breakdown of the blood-brain barrier (BBB) • Infertility • Several neurological effects including depression[116] • Sleep disruption • Cataracts • Neural development and autism[117]

The ultimate proof that Pall's work is not just theory is that multiple studies have shown that the VGCCs-disrupting effects of EMFs can be stopped just by taking calcium blockers, which prevent calcium from flowing into the cells. But don't start popping pills just yet... we'll get into EMF-protection solutions soon enough.

3. EMFs Open Up Your Body's Barriers Against Toxic Invaders

"The most important [effect from EMFs] is the opening of the blood–brain barrier. This allows mercury, organochlorines and other pollutants to enter the brain, where they cause various neurodegenerative diseases."

- French oncologist Dominique Belpomme[118]

---

112 ncbi.nlm.nih.gov/pubmed/22005645
113 sites.google.com
114 As reported by Dr. Elizabeth Plourde in *EMF Freedom*. See ncbi.nlm.nih.gov/pubmed/15225800
115 Idem. See journals.plos.org/plosone/article?id=10.1371/journal.pone.0047429
116 researchgate.net
117 See Martin Pall's presentation on the subject: youtube.com/watch?v=yydZZanRJ50
118 emfacts.com

Allan Frey — the biologist I told you about in Chapter 2 — first proved that low level of EMF radiation (like those emitted by a smartphone) can open the important barrier which protects your brain from toxins and other invaders, AKA "the blood-brain barrier", or BBB for short.

As Martin Blank reports:[119]

"Frey was interested in whether EMF exposure would impair the BBB. He studied two sets of rats: One set, which he exposed to 1.9 GHz radiation (comparable to a cell phone) for two hours and a second set, which did not receive that radiation exposure.

First, he injected a fluorescent dye into the circulatory system of each unexposed rat. As expected, the dye spread very quickly into all the tissues except the brain. Then he injected the same dye into the exposed rats, and within a matter of minutes from this single exposure the dye had leached into the brain."

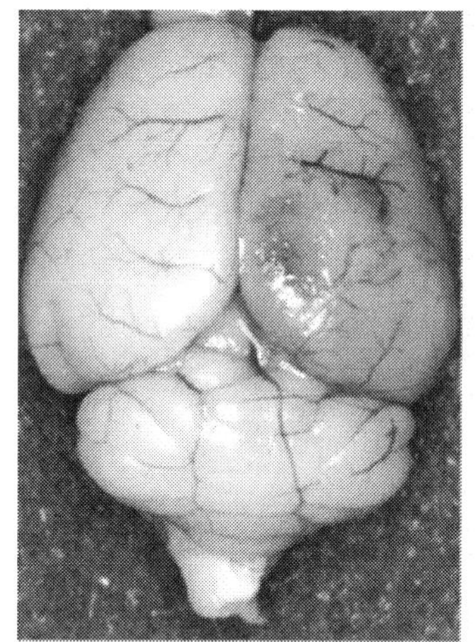

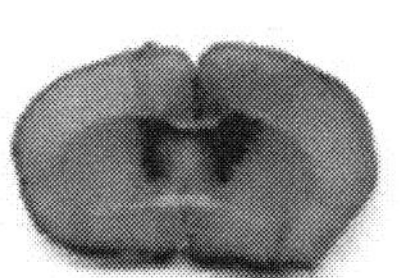

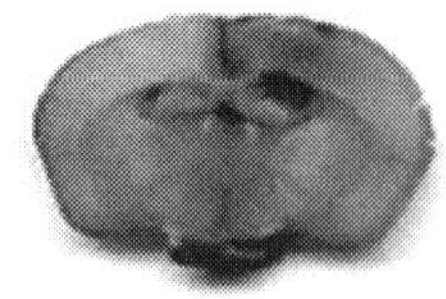

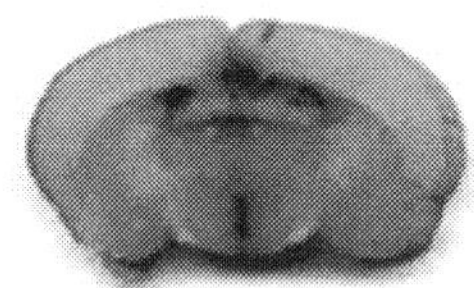

In a classic fashion, Frey's career was cut short when he proved that this non-ionizing radiation caused harm to rats. Fortunately, his results have been confirmed by a lot of other researchers, including:

- Professor Leif Salford in Sweden[120]
- Nora Volkow, MD and director of the National Institute on Drug Abuse[121]
- Triple-doctorate[122] and Polish researcher Dariusz Leszczynski[123]

---

119 Blank, M., PhD. (2015). *Overpowered: The Dangers of Electromagnetic Radiation (EMF) and What You Can Do about It.* Seven Stories Press.
120 portal.research.lu.se
121 ncbi.nlm.nih.gov/pmc/articles/PMC3184892
122 gigahertz.ch
123 ncbi.nlm.nih.gov/pubmed/12076339

Effects Of BBB Leakage	
Positive	**Negative**
• Drug delivery in the brain[124] • Potential applications to treat brain tumors[125]	• Headaches or migraines[126] • Death of some brain cells[127] • Allows viruses, heavy metals and bacteria to break into the brain • Disrupts nerve cells and overall brain function • Damage to the nervous system,[128] increased symptoms of neurodegenerative diseases like Alzheimer's or MS • Memory loss[129] • Increased demand in glucose (sugar) from the brain

This BBB leakage seems to be triggered very quickly by the use of a cell phone. In one study, women whose blood was drawn right after a short phone call showed higher levels of a specific thyroid hormone carrier — the proof that their cerebrospinal fluid was leaking in their blood.[130]

The most concerning part is that this damage may last for days, if not weeks. In Salford's research, rats exposed to cell phone radiation for just 2 hours still had a leaking BBB 8 weeks after the exposure.

This BBB leakage has also been found in people exposed to high levels of Dirty Electricity (DE). When epidemiologist Samuel Milham and electrician Dave Stetzer reduced the DE levels in a public library from 10,000 GS units (extreme concern level) to under 50 GS units (safety threshold) using special filters, they found out that the urine levels of neurotransmitters in participants who worked there decreased immensely.[131]

---

124 ncbi.nlm.nih.gov/pmc/articles/PMC5858162

125 Dr. Frank S. Lieberman has recently developed a device which uses low level EMFs to treat brain tumors. This device has been approved by the FDA and has been shown to be more effective than many chemotherapy drugs in treating specific types of brain tumors. See his presentation here: youtube.com/watch?v=ugDkVSuiPtg

126 As reported by Dr. Elizabeth Plourde in *EMF Freedom*. See ncbi.nlm.nih.gov/pmc/articles/PMC1533043/

127 As reported by Dr. Martin Blank in *Overpowered*. See ncbi.nlm.nih.gov/pubmed/19345073

128 As reported by Dr. Elizabeth Plourde in *EMF Freedom*. See hindawi.com/journals/np/2015/708306/

129 Idem. See ncbi.nlm.nih.gov/pubmed/25598203

130 Idem. See ehjournal.biomedcentral.com/articles/10.1186/1476-069X-8-19

131 stetzerelectric.com

This matches all the observations I've talked about above, which indicate that EMFs open up your BBB and let the bad stuff in (toxins) while leaking the good stuff out (nutrients, neurotransmitters).

Independent researchers also argue we should consider the possibility that EMFs could be contributing to the weakening of other important barriers in the human body, including:[132]

- The blood-ocular barrier (protects the eyes) — links with cataracts and myopia
- The blood-placenta barrier (protects the developing fetus) — links with fetal problems in children, autism and miscarriages
- The blood-gut barrier (protects proper digestion and nutrition) — links with autoimmune diseases, food intolerance, digestive disorders, Lyme disease symptoms
- The blood-testes barrier (protects developing sperm) — links with infertility, loss of libido, cancer, impotency

I personally think our EMF exposure might be one of the many reasons we see such an increase in digestive autoimmune diseases like celiac and Crohn's, food allergies and digestive disorders like IBS — which are all linked with intestinal permeability,[133] AKA "leaky gut syndrome". I guess the future will tell.

4. EMFs Reduce Your Body's Ability To Heal

"If you are in any way concerned about your well-being, then dealing with nighttime exposures to EMFs is the absolute foundation on which you can build a healthy life."

- Lloyd Burrell, former electro-hypersensitivity (EHS) sufferer and founder of ElectricSense.com

In what seems to be a serious episode of bad karma, EMFs not only seem to damage the DNA of your cells, make them overflow with calcium and leave your body's natural barriers wide open to toxins and invaders — they also prevent your body from healing and repairing this damage.

It's a known fact that nighttime is when most of your body heals itself from everything you throw at it during the day. The second you fall asleep, your body follows a very specific detoxification schedule, including:

- Your brain cells shrink by around 60%[134] to allow your glymphatic system — which was discovered just a few years ago — to take the garbage (toxins and metabolites) out[135]

132 bioinitiative.org
133 ncbi.nlm.nih.gov/pmc/articles/PMC4253991
134 mercola.com
135 nih.gov

- Events of the day get stored in your long-term memory[136]
- Your body does most of its autophagy — an essential process which gets rid of useless or damaged cells
- Your muscles and tissues get repaired[137]

Spending as much time as possible in the most restorative sleep stage called "R.E.M. sleep" is particularly important. A good indication that your body spends time in this restorative stage is that you're able to recall your dreams. If you're like most people I talk to, this very rarely happens.[138]

The most important way high levels of EMFs in your bedroom environment can impair your healing ability is by disrupting your melatonin hormone production.

As explains Martin Blank,[139] by 2000 there were already 15 different studies demonstrating that Magnetic Fields, Electric Fields and RF radiation suppress your body's ability to produce melatonin. Less melatonin rhymes with less REM sleep, and less healing.[140]

This effect has been shown in a dose-response manner — the more EMFs you're exposed to, the more your melatonin gets suppressed.[141]

And don't start thinking you're all good if you just avoid using your cell phone right before getting your ZZZs on. One study showed that using your cell phone for just 25 minutes during the day will significantly reduce the amount of melatonin your body produces at night.

Just in case you need more evidence that EMFs impair sleep, here's one more.

A few years ago, Prof Trevor Marshall from the Autoimmunity Research Foundation wanted to prove that sleeping in a very low EMF environment could improve sleep. He asked a bunch of people to sleep in a weird but very effective anti-EMF "sleeping bag" which completely covered participants during the night — leaving an opening for the eyes, nose and mouth.[142] The results? 90% of them

136 ncbi.nlm.nih.gov/pmc/articles/PMC3783537
137 sleepfoundation.org
138 huffingtonpost.com
139 Blank, M., PhD. (2015). *Overpowered: The Dangers of Electromagnetic Radiation (EMF) and What You Can Do about It*. Seven Stories Press.
140 academic.oup.com
141 As reported by Dr. Martin Blank in *Overpowered*. See microwavenews.com/news/backissues/n-d97issue.pdf
142 stopumts.nl

reported sleeping much better.[143]

Can EMFs Affect Sleep?[144]

Studies	RF Radiation (V/m)	Effects
A	0.047-0.22	↑ Fatigue & Sleep Disorders
B	0.14	↑ Sleep Disturbances
C	0.19-0.64	↑ Fatigue & Sleep Disorders
D	0.19-0.43	↑ Sleep Disturbances
E	0.43-0.61	↑ Fatigue & Sleep Disorders
F	13.72	↓ REM Sleep
FCC Limit	61.4	

Studies	RF Radiation (SAR W/kg)	Effects
G	0.25	↓ REM Sleep
H	1	↓ Sleep Quality
I	1	↓ Sleep Quality
J	1	↓ Sleep Quality
K	1	↓ Sleep Quality
FCC Limit	1.6	FCC Limit
L	1.95	↓REM Sleep
M	2	↓ Sleep Quality

Aside from reducing your sleep quality, EMFs also might prevent your cells from healing in multiple other ways:

- **EMFs reduce your body's reserves of two key antioxidants** — superoxide dismutase and glutathione peroxidase.[145] Less antioxidant power, less healing.

143 Discussion between Lloyd Burrell and Prof Trevor Marshall, as part of ElectricSense.com's EMF Experts Solutions Club. See electricsense.com for more details.
144 List of detailed references available in Annex 1.
145 As reported by Daniel and Ryan DeBaun in *Radiation Nation*. See ncbi.nlm.nih.gov/pmc/articles/PMC4344711/

- **EMFs make your red blood cells (RBC) clump together**[146] which reduces oxygen delivery throughout your whole body. Less oxygen, less healing.[147]

- **EMFs increase your cortisol levels — a key stress hormone.**[148] More cortisol, slower healing.[149]

The Tip Of The Iceberg

At this point, there are already enough black swan studies that show that EMFs can have serious biological effects — both positive and negative — at levels sometimes thousands of times lower than the current safety guidelines.

What does it all mean for your own health though? Can we blame invisible EMFs for specific diseases, certain health symptoms you might be experiencing?

Let's dive into the uncertainty and see...

146 youtube.com
147 ncbi.nlm.nih.gov/pmc/articles/PMC2704021
148 According to Olga Sheean, even short-term exposure to radiation from a cell phone tower has been shown to increase cortisol levels, with long-term exposure resulting in permanently elevated adrenaline. See the German study here: avaate.org/IMG/pdf/Rimbach-Study-20112.pdf
149 ncbi.nlm.nih.gov/pubmed/15110929

Chapter 5

THE NOT-SO-EVIDENT

135 "Black Swan" Studies

Is Electrosensitivity Real?

8 Ways EMFs *Might* Affect You

What We Don't Know For Sure (Yet)

It ain't what you don't know that gets you into trouble.
It's what you know for sure that just ain't so.

- Mark Twain, of course... Every good book contains a Mark Twain quote.

In March 2016, the city of Berkeley in California passed the "Right-To-Know Ordinance" which "requires wireless retailers to warn customers of possible radiation exposure when purchasing cell phones."[150]

While some people think this is totally crazy,[151] I honestly think it's only fair considering the fact that manufacturers themselves are giving their customers the laughable advice to never to hold a smartphone near your body, and that our EMF standards are based on completely outdated heating effects, not biological effects.

In the last chapter, I showed you a bunch of possible ways EMFs can disrupt key processes inside each one of your cells, and hopefully I didn't bore you to death with the lingo.

The real question is... what direct or indirect side effects could EMFs have on your health, especially considering the fact that the EMF soup we live in is getting thicker and thicker?

135 Studies (And One Nosebleed) Later...

You've probably heard a thousand times that cell phones might be linked with brain or breast cancer. But let me tell you, it's only the tip of the iceberg.

Digging through the research of the top EMF experts on the planet, I found out that EMFs could be affecting your health on so many levels — including your sleep, hormones, mood, weight loss (or gain), mental clarity, and much, much more.

---

150 rfsafe.com

151 Like the telecom industry, who has been suing the city of Berkeley over this labeling: sanfrancisco.cbslocal.com/2017/02/24/judge-orders-california-to-release-papers-discussing-risk-of-cell-phone-use/

Out of the thousands I gathered during my research, I picked 135 papers that show links between EMF exposure and certain adverse health effects — a vast majority of which happens at levels below the current safety limits. Each one of these studies is a "black swan" which shatters the idea that EMFs cannot possibly affect you outside the heating effects.

Does this mean that EMFs are the cause of all these chronic diseases and health issues? Of course not. But even if there's a slight chance they may affect your health, I'm sure you'll want to hear about it.

Warnings were put on cigarettes decades before we finally proved they cause cancer. Who knows which warnings are going to appear on the iPhone 10?[152]

152 In *EMF Freedom*, Elizabeth & Marcus Plourde talked about every possible consequence which can happen when you mess with human cells the way our EMF soup does — and argued that each one of these health effects could eventually appear as warnings on smartphone labels. The next part is highly inspired from their work — without which none of this would have been possible.

Warning #1: EMFs Might Make You Sick

Estimated prevalence of self-proclaimed electro-hypersensitivity (EHS) in various countries[153]

Prevalence of EHS	Country	Year Of Survey
1.5%[154]	Sweden	1997
3.2%[155]	United States	1998
5%[156]	Switzerland	2004
9%[157]	Germany	2004
11%[158]	England	2004
13.3%[159]	Taiwan	2007
No one knows!	Worldwide	2030

Throughout the world, reports of people claiming to be sensitive to EMFs from smartphones, smart meters or even just standard household electricity are appearing by the thousands.

Scratch that. According to research by Magda Havas, PhD, the real number of people showing signs of *extreme* electro-hypersensitivity (or "EHS") might be around 25 million, while 300 million more people might have moderate symptoms "like headaches or difficulty sleeping."[160]

A lot of medical professionals are also seeing this concerning trend. In 2016, about a third of all doctors in the Netherlands had been contacted by someone who said they suffered because of EMFs.[161]

So... are all these people crazy and suddenly went full woo-woo?

---

153 Based on the investigations of Havas (2013 — semanticscholar.org), Hallberg and Oberfeld (2006 — next-up.org) and Hedendahl, Carlberg & Hardell (2015 — researchgate.net)
154 ncbi.nlm.nih.gov/pubmed/11871850
155 ncbi.nlm.nih.gov/pmc/articles/PMC1241215
156 ncbi.nlm.nih.gov/pubmed/17193782
157 bmub.bund.de
158 who.int
159 ncbi.nlm.nih.gov/pubmed/21982467
160 semanticscholar.org
161 ncbi.nlm.nih.gov/pubmed/27939136

The Swedish Government doesn't think so — and has been recognizing EHS as a functional impairment (AKA not a delusional mental disease) since... wait for it... 1995.[162] Geez.

What do the Swedes know that we just don't get? Why are "science-based medicine" proponents still clinging to the idea that EHS is a mental disease?[163] I honestly have no idea, but the word "denial" comes to mind.

Seriously, one of the reasons is probably that the exact definition of EHS is very unclear and that different people get different symptoms from different lengths of exposure to different kinds of EMF signals.

Most Common Symptoms Of EHS[164]

Skin problems	Sensitivity to light/eye problems	Tiredness / weakness
Heart problems / high blood pressure	Headaches / migraine	Pain in joints / muscles
Dizziness	Concentration difficulties	Nausea / general poor health
Endocrine reactions	Memory disorders	Respiratory / lung disorders
Stomach / intestinal disorders	Numbness	"Influenza" / throat problems
Sleep disorders	Hearing problems/tinnitus	Tremors/cramps
Anxiety/depression	Haziness/confusion	Fainting/coma
Asthma/allergies	Speech difficulties	Irritability

As you can see, there are so many symptoms related to EHS that could also be caused by diet, exercise, meds or a thousand of other factors.

This leads us to a bunch of very important questions we all need to ask ourselves like... am I irritable because of EMFs, or because I'm having a bad day? Is my digestion poor because of EMFs, or because I ate something my body simply doesn't agree with?

I could go on and on, but you get the point — it's hard to say if your health symptoms are directly *caused* by EMFs, *aggravated* by EMFs, or just caused by something else. And once you start learning the truth about EMFs just like you're doing at this very moment, it's easy to start blaming

162 eloverkanslig.org
163 sciencebasedmedicine.org
164 Results of a Swedish study looking at the symptoms of over 400 EHS sufferers. See feb.se/feb/blackonwhite-complete-book.pdf

everything on these invisible signals — and automatically come off as one of those "crazy tinfoils".

In order to really know whether your body is sensitive to EMFs or not, we'd have to look at how it's affecting something scientifically *tangible* and *measurable* — like the biomarkers in your blood. And are there credible studies which show that people who claim they're sensitive to EMFs have the screwed up biomarkers to show for it? You bet.

In a 2015 article published in *Reviews on Environmental Health*, "scientists who have been studying 700 electromagnetic sensitive, as well as multiple chemically sensitive people, since 2009 found that chronic inflammation was the key process for the development of [EHS]."[165]

People who said they were electro-sensitive indeed had increased levels of histamine (high in those suffering from allergies), anti-myelin antibodies (linked with muscle weakness and tingling sensations), decreased melatonin (linked with insomnia and reduced immunity) and oxidative stress (linked to basically every disease known to man). More importantly, researchers found the exact same biomarkers in animals exposed EMFs.

Still think it's "all in their head"? Let me show you more, and you be the judge...

In 2002, a study by researcher Santini and his colleagues[166] surveyed 270 men and 260 women who lived at different distances from a cell phone base station (tower).

Their work confirmed a pretty obvious hypothesis: the closer people lived to a powerful cell phone tower blasting their body with RF radiation 24/7, the more EHS-related symptoms they experienced — including fatigue, poor sleep, headaches, a feeling of discomfort, difficulty concentrating, depression and memory loss.[167]

---

165 As reported by Dr. Elizabeth Plourde in *EMF Freedom*.
See emfacts.com/2016/01/ehs-paper-published-in-reviews-on-environmental-health/

166 ncbi.nlm.nih.gov/pubmed/12168254

167 As reported by Magda Havas, PhD, in
https://www.semanticscholar.org/paper/Radiation-from-wireless-technology-affects-the-the-Havas/38a99baa23f295f886f25f5784ea6f9c31ee5232

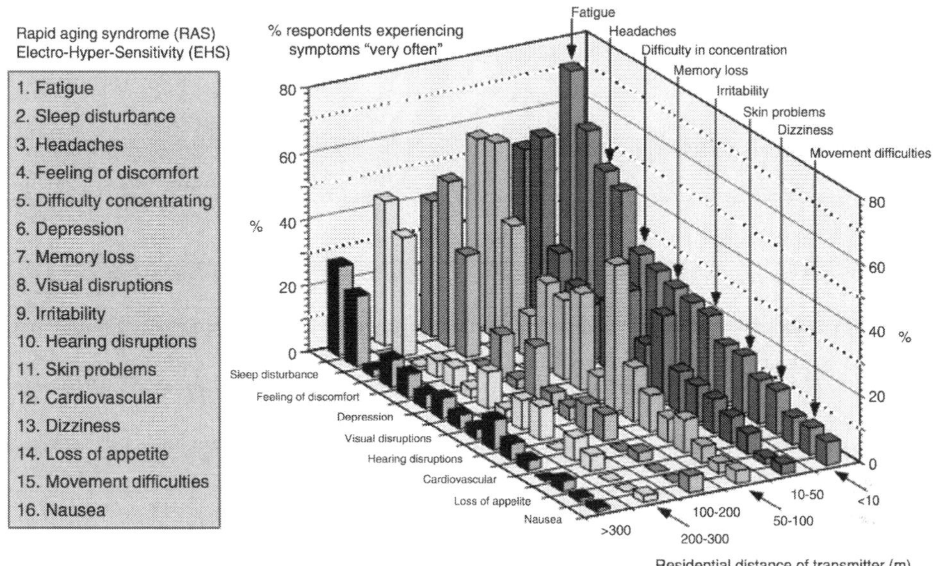

Symptoms experienced by people near cellular phone base stations. Based on the work of Santini et al., and reproduced with the permission of Magda Havas, PhD.

The researchers concluded that people shouldn't live within 300 meters of a cellular tower. Now this might be a problem, because 15 years after this study the number of base stations around the world has... how can I put this... "skyrocketed":

Cellular Towers & Wifi Networks Worldwide, 2002-2003[168]

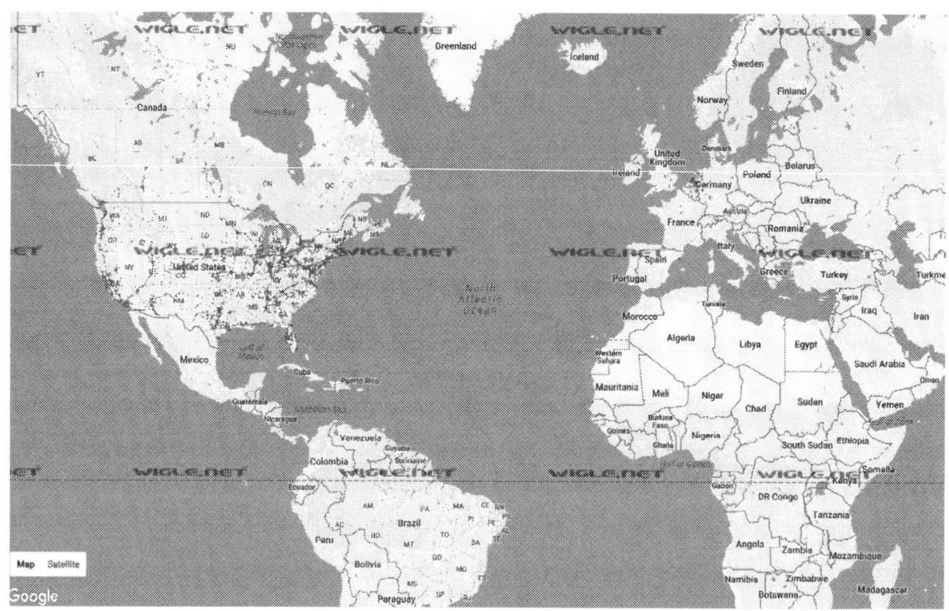

Cellular Towers & Wifi Networks Worldwide, 2016-2017[169]

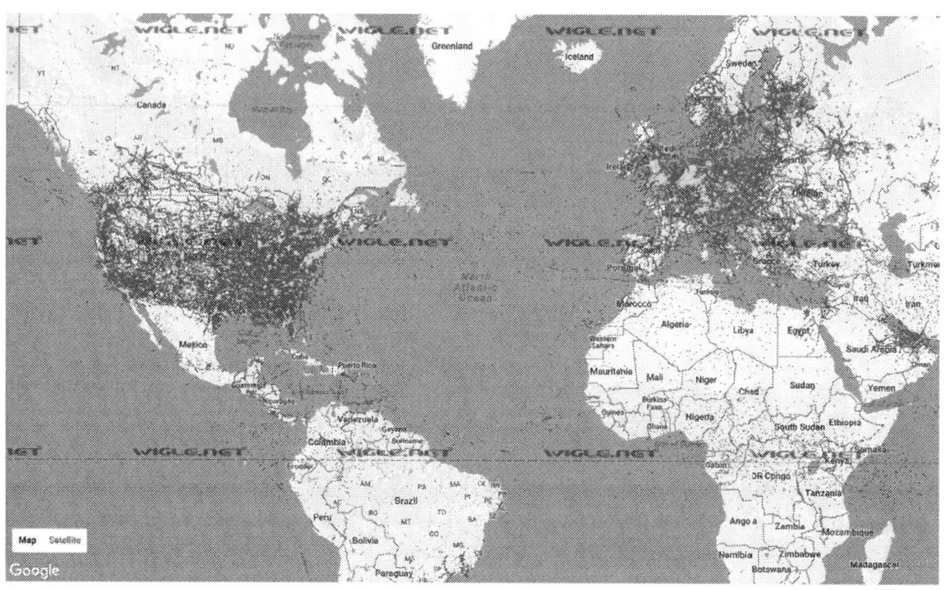

168 Generated using Wigle.net on 04/19/17. Although I can't guarantee its accuracy, this map does give you a fair idea of how much our EMF soup has changed in just a few years.

169 Idem.

EMFs are pretty much like coffee. Everyone is sensitive to caffeine, but to different degrees — some people get so jittery and energized, and some people can down 3 cups of coffee before bed and sleep just fine. And I think everyone is affected by EMFs, but some more than others.

Want to figure out if *you* are sensitive to EMFs? Try putting your 4G cell phone right on your nightstand while you sleep for 3 straight days — then spend 3 days sleeping with the same phone next to your head, but on "airplane mode". And repeat the experiment multiple times to be 100% sure you're not making this all up.

If you wake up more refreshed or are able to recall your dreams better (signs of deep REM sleep) when your cell phone isn't blasting your head with RF radiation... welcome to the club of "EMF-sensitive" people!

Warning #2: EMFs Might Increase Your Cancer Risks

Can EMFs Affect Brain Cancer Risks?[170]

Findings	Study
Increased risk of brain tumors, especially on the same side	Bortkiewicz et al., 2017
Increased risk of brain tumors	Myung et al., 2009
Increased risk of brain tumours especially in long-term users (≥10 years)	Prasad et al., 2017
Increased risks of glioma	Carlberg and Hardell, 2012
Possible association between heavy mobile phone use and brain tumors	Coureau et al., 2014
Occupational magnetic field exposure increases the risk of glioblastoma	Villeneuve et al., 2002
Glioma and acoustic neuroma should be considered to be caused by EMF emissions from cell phones	Carlberg and Hardell, 2013
Mobile phone radiation causes brain tumors and should be classified as a probable human carcinogen (Class 2A)	Morgan et al., 2015

Can EMFs Affect Breast Cancer Risks?[171]

Findings	Study
Increased risk of breast cancer in radio operators	Tynes et al., 1996
Women under 50 were 7X more likely to develop oestrogen receptor-positive breast cancer when exposed to magnetic field levels over 1 mG	Feychting et al., 1998
Plausible link between EMF and breast cancer	Caplan et al., 2000
Occupational exposure to magnetic fields over 25 mG increases risks of breast cancer by 3-fold	Forssén et al., 2000
Cluster of male breast cancer in office workers exposed to high levels of magnetic fields	Milham, 2004
Long-term significant occupational exposure to ELF MF may certainly increase the risk of both Alzheimer's disease and breast cancer	Davanipour and Sobel, 2009
Possible link between magnetic fields exposure and breast cancer	Chen et al., 2013
EMF exposure may be associated with the increase risk of male breast cancer	Sun et al., 2013
Low levels of magnetic fields increase risks of breast cancer	Zhao et al., 2014

170 List of detailed references available in Annex 2.
171 List of detailed references available in Annex 3.

In 2011, the International Agency For Research On Cancer (IARC) — which is part of the World Health Organization — classified EMFs as a class 2B "possible" carcinogen.[172]
Then, somewhere in the last years, they edited the entire discourse on their website from "EMFs might cause cancer" to just "cell phone radiation might cause cancer".[173] Odd, if I may say so myself.

Either way, this puts EMFs or RF radiation from cell phones in the same category as DDT (pesticide banned since 1972[174]), lead, and diesel fuel.

Is that a sufficient argument to conclude EMFs might increase your cancer risks? After all, in that same class 2B carcinogen category you can find stuff most would consider "superfoods" like Aloe Vera, Ginkgo biloba extract and... pickled veggies.[175]

But this IARC classification was not a fluke, and the results of the NTP study I've told you about in Chapter 3 pretty much put the nail in the skeptics' coffin — showing that just 30 minutes of cell phone use per day for 36 years can significantly increase your risks of glioma (a kind of brain tumor) and schwannoma (a rare kind of heart tumor).[176]

But this is not the first time different types of EMFs have been linked with increased risks of various cancers.

In 1979 — way before any smartphone or cell tower started exposing us to RF radiation — researchers were starting to establish a link between high levels of Magnetic Fields (MF) from standard household wiring or high-voltage power lines and childhood leukemia.[177] In 2002, this actually lead IARC to slap these 50-60 Hz MF fields with a Class 2B category too.[178]

Since then, dozens of studies have linked EMFs and many other different types of cancer including

172 iarc.fr
173 Discussion between Lloyd Burrell and Girish Kumar, PhD, from the Indian Institute of Technology Bombay, as part of ElectricSense.com's EMF Experts Solutions Club. See IARC's official website which now talks about "cell phone radiation might cause cancer": who.int/mediacentre/factsheets/fs193/en/
174 npic.orst.edu
175 en.wikipedia.org
176 microwavesnews.com
177 ncbi.nlm.nih.gov/pubmed/453167
178 jstor.org

melanoma (skin cancer),[179] acoustic neuroma (inner ear),[180] breast cancer,[181] salivary gland cancer[182] and lymphoma (white blood cells)[183] — just to name these few.

The most concerning part here in my humble opinion is that there's no way to know how much our current 2017 EMF soup will impact your cancer risks later in life, considering that certain tumors take decades to develop. Hiroshima survivors, for example, are still seeing increases in brain tumors more than 65 years after having been exposed to radiation.[184]

But focusing on cancer research to determine whether EMFs are dangerous or not is seriously nuts — because most of it comes down to counting body bags, figuring out who died of brain tumors and how much they used their phone, and possibly end up saying "oops, we're sorry about that".

179 researchgate.net
180 As reported by Daniel and Ryan DeBaun in *Radiation Nation*. See pathophysiologyjournal.com/article/S0928-4680(14)00064-9/fulltext
181 Idem. See ncbi.nlm.nih.gov/pubmed/24984538
182 academic.oup.com
183 sfdph.org
184 nytimes.com

Warning #3: EMFs Might Screw Up Your Male Hormones, Sperm Quality & Sex Drive

Can EMFs Affect Men's Fertility?[185]

Studies	RF Radiation (V/m)	Effects
A	0.036	↓ Sperm Count
B	0.5-0.6	↓ Sperm Morphology
C	0.79-2	↑ Irreversible Infertility
D	1.37	↑ Damage In Testes
E	1.37-1.94	↓ Sperm Motility
F	43.41	↓ Testosterone
FCC Limit	61.4	FCC Limit

Studies	RF Radiation (SAR W/kg)	Effects
G	0.0024	↓ Sperm Morphology
H	0.0071	↑ Damage In Testes
I	0.091	↑ Damage In Testes
J	0.4	↓ Sperm Motility
K	1.2	↑ Damage In Testes
L	1.46	↓ Sperm Motility
FCC Limit	1.6	FCC Limit
M	2	↓ Sperm Morphology

Guys, you need to hear about the new, amazing contraceptive in town. It's effective, free, and you won't even feel it!

It's called "blasting your crotch with RF radiation by keeping your smartphone in your pocket (like 67% of all Canadian adults do)[186] or using a laptop on your lap".

185 List of detailed references available in Annex 4.
186 Statistic cited in this exposé by CBC's Marketplace. See youtube.com/watch?v=Wm69ik_Qdb8&app=desktop

Can EMFs Affect Men's Fertility? (Meta-Analyses)[187]

Year Of Publication	# Of Studies Looked At	Conclusion	Study
2014	10	Mobile phone exposure negatively affects sperm quality.	Adams et al., 2014
2012	26	Sperm exposed to RF radiation show decreased motility, morphometric abnormalities, and increased oxidative stress, whereas men using mobile phones have decreased sperm concentration, decreased motility and decreased viability.	La Vignera et al., 2012
2009	99	RF from cell phones might affect the fertilizing potential of spermatozoa.	Desai et al., 2009
2013	11	Mobile phone radiation has a tendency to significantly affect sperm quality.	Dama and Bhat, 2013
2014	18	Evidence from current studies suggests potential harmful effects of mobile phone use on semen parameters.	Liu et al., 2014
2016	27	RF is able to induce mitochondrial dysfunction [in sperm] leading to oxidative stress.	Houston et al., 2016

Okay, maybe infertility is not something to laugh at, but what can I tell you — humor is my coping mechanism. The fact is that a whole lot of young couples these days are unable to conceive naturally — about half of them in the city of Mumbai, India.[188]

There are very good reasons to think this huge drop in fertility, libido, sperm count, testosterone and every other aspect of male reproductive health can be linked to our increasing EMF exposure.

EMFs & Sperm Count: As reported by Daniel DeBaun in *Radiation Nation*, "Research has shown that using a laptop directly in the lap, especially in conjunction with Wifi, is associated with a decrease in sperm count and motility while causing sperm DNA damage".[189]

Multiple studies have concluded the exact same thing — one Argentinian paper showing that using

187 List of detailed references available in Annex 5.
188 According to Girish Kumar, PhD, from the Indian Institute of Technology Bombay.
189 As reported by Daniel and Ryan DeBaun in *Radiation Nation*. See ncbi.nlm.nih.gov/pubmed/18044740

your laptop for 4 hours can make 25% of your spermatozoids basically useless.[190]

Other studies have found similar sperm damage from cell phone use. In one study, heavy cell phone users (4+ hours per day) had a 40% lower sperm count compared to people who didn't use a cell phone.[191]

And in case you personally couldn't care less about your sperm count because you already have enough children or have no plans of having children soon... it's good to know that your sperm quality is closely linked to your overall health.

A Danish investigation found that "men with the highest sperm counts enjoyed a mortality rate 43% lower than the men with the lowest counts."[192]

EMFs & Testosterone: Studies are limited on the subject, but one study found that "exposing rats to the cell phone frequency of 900 MHz for 2 hours a day for 45 days leads to a reduction in their testosterone levels. Exposed rats had testosterone levels of 176 ng/dl compared to the non-exposed rats levels averaging 505 ng/dl."[193]

I think it's reasonable to hypothesize that anything which affects your testes and reduces your sperm quality can possibly affect your production of sexual hormones like testosterone as well. One study did show that exposure to cell phone radiation during pregnancy in rats could cause offsprings to suffer from oxidative damage to the testicles, resulting in early puberty.[194]

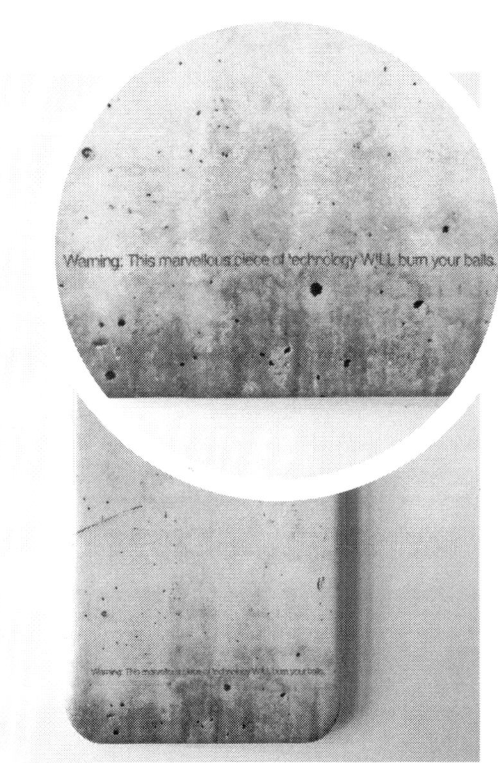

May I never forget the wise advice I've engraved on my iPhone case. It reads: "Warning: This marvellous piece of technology WILL burn your balls."

190 Idem. See dx.doi.org/10.1016/j.fertnstert.2011.10.012
191 As reported by Dr. Martin Blank in *Overpowered*. See ncbi.nlm.nih.gov/pubmed/17482179
192 health.harvard.edu
193 As reported by Dr. Elizabeth Plourde in *EMF Freedom*. See ncbi.nlm.nih.gov/labs/articles/22897402/
194 Idem. See ncbi.nlm.nih.gov/pubmed/24101576

EMFs & Erectile Dysfunction: As Daniel DeBaun explains, cell phones might also be part of the reason sales of Viagra and Cialis have been soaring: "In 2013, researchers found links between cell phone use and erectile dysfunction. Subsequent large-scale studies have confirmed the initial data and have compelled scientists to recommend exploring the mechanisms involved in this phenomenon."[195]

195 As reported by Daniel and Ryan DeBaun in *Radiation Nation*. See ncbi.nlm.nih.gov/pmc/articles/PMC3921848/

Warning #4: EMFs Might Screw Up Your Female Hormones & Sex Drive... And Trigger Early Menopause

Headaches, depression, disrupted cycle, insomnia, the feeling that you might strangle someone if they even remotely say between the lines that you're going nuts... is it early menopause, or is it something else?

In a 2015 interview, Alternative medicine practitioner and author of *EMF Freedom* Elizabeth Plourde shares that she found a strong link between EMFs and what her patients *thought* were symptoms of menopause:

"[The problem] wasn't hormones on any of these women. So I spoke to each one, really in depth. What's different, what's new, what has changed that you're feeling like this? And the common denominator was that they had had a smart meter, the electrical smart meter that they're now measuring electricity with across the nation and in other countries in the world too."[196]

Does that mean EMFs are solely responsible for all your hormonal problems? Probably not. But they probably are making matters worse — as a lot of studies demonstrate.

EMFs & Female Hormones: Women need some testosterone too, so this means EMFs can probably affect them just as much as men. In a study looking at "180 female workers exposed to EMFs for 1 year compared to 349 controls, researchers found the radiation led to a significant increase in menstrual disorders, increased menorrhagia (heavy bleeding), and a reduction in progesterone levels."[197]

EMFs & Uterine Health: Sorry ladies, but it's not because you don't have delicate sperms to take care of that you should use your laptop on your lap or keep your cell phone in your pocket.

Unsurprisingly, exposing your groin to a 900 MHZ mobile phone signal has been shown to induce endometrial impairment, creating damage at both the biochemical and histological cellular levels.[198]

And while men can completely renew their sperm reserve in just 74 days,[199] the 300,000 potential eggs you get from birth are not considered to be renewable. The latest research has even shown that most women have less than 12% of this egg pool left by age 30, and less than 3% by age 40.[200]

196 ihealthtube.com
197 As reported by Elizabeth Plourde in *EMF Freedom*. See ncbi.nlm.nih.gov/pubmed/18771615
198 Idem. See ncbi.nlm.nih.gov/pubmed/18536493
199 ncbi.nlm.nih.gov/pmc/articles/PMC4698398
200 telegraph.co.uk

EMFs & Female Fertility: If EMFs generally prevent your body from repairing itself and cause damage and stress to your cells, it's logical they could also be disrupting female fertility just as much as male fertility when you seriously expose your reproductive organs.

As reported by epidemiologist Sam Milham in his latest book,[201] electrician Dave Stetzer visited a bank where many women clerks "were having difficulty getting pregnant or were suffering spontaneous abortions".

He examined the bank, found high levels of Dirty Electricity, and reduced these levels dramatically using special filters. A year or so later he got an angry call from the bank manager, complaining that many of his workers had left simultaneously on maternity leave."

---

201 Milham, S., MD. (2012). *Dirty Electricity: Electrification and the Diseases of Civilization*. iUniverse

Warning #5: EMFs Might Be Messing With Your Head

Can EMFs Affect Your Head?[202]

Studies	RF Radiation (V/m)	Effects
A	0.14-0.39	↑ Headaches
B	0.15	↑ Behavioral Problems
C	0.24-0.89	↓ Calmness
D	0.55	↓ Memory
E	0.7	↓ Cognition
F	0.78	↑ Behavioral Problems
G	0.89-2.19	↑ Headaches
H	1.74-6.14	↑ Behavioral Problems
I	1.94	↑ Blood-Brain Barrier Leakage
J	2.37	↓ Memory
K	8.68	↓ Neurotransmitters
L	11.07-12.85	↑ Oxidative Stress On Cornea
M	13-34	↑ Oxidative Stress In Brain
N	14.31	↑ Oxidative Stress In Brain
O	15.14	↓ Neurotransmitters
FCC Limit	61.4	FCC Limit
P	62.6	↑ Oxidative Stress In Brain

202 List of detailed references available in Annex 6.

Studies	RF Radiation (SAR W/kg)	Effects
Q	0.00067	↓ Memory, Learning
R	0.0016 - 0.0044	↑ Behavioral Problems
S	0.016-2	↓ Neuron Formation
T	0.17-0.58	↑ Oxidative Stress In Brain
U	0.31-0.78	↑ Oxidative Stress In Bone Marrow
V	0.37	↑ Oxidative Stress In Brain
W	0.41-0.98	↑ Impaired Memory In Rats
X	1.38-1.45	↑ Neurotoxic Biomarkers
Y	1.5	↑ Oxidative Stress In Brain
Z	1.51	↑ DNA Damage
AA	1.6	↑ DNA Damage In Human Hair
BB	Smartphone 6h/d	↑ Allergy Symptoms
CC	Computer 8h/d	↑ Oxidative Stress In Eyes
FCC Limit	1.6	FCC Limit

If EMFs coming off a smartphone are so strongly linked with an increased risk of brain tumors, the next question that comes to mind is... what else can it do to your head?

The problem is that your skull is not some kind of incredible anti-EMF protective shell — and that radiation does get into certain areas of your head when you call someone to tell them how bored you are, or even spend all day next to a wifi router.

There's great evidence that just a couple of minutes per day of this RF exposure can have serious effects on your mood, memory, eyes and ears — at levels below the FCC "safety" guidelines, of course.

EMFs & Your Mood

EMFs might seriously affect your mood — and not just when the wifi at Starbucks is so slow that you suddenly feel like you're back on an old school 56k dial up modem.

As reported by EMF activist Olga Sheean,[203] "German psychiatrist Dr. Christine Aschermann reports seeing multiple effects on the brain, with an 'increased occurrence of cognitive and psychological disorders with exposure to telecommunications'."[204]

In his 2015 paper, researcher Martin Pall, PhD, (remember, the excess calcium/VGCCs guy?) has reviewed dozens of studies and found "26 studies associated [EMFs] with neuropsychiatric effects, with 5 criteria showing causality".[205]

In the worst cases, some researchers have concluded that EMF exposure might be linked with an increase in anxiety (by depleting your brain of a neurotransmitter called "GABA"[206]), depression[207] and even suicidal thoughts.[208]

Again, this doesn't necessarily mean that using your cell phone will automatically make you depressed or nuts. But there's a very strong chance that opening up your blood-brain barrier, depleting your brain from its neurotransmitters, causing excess calcium to flow into your cells and causing direct DNA damage to your neurons might all be taking away a chunk of your happiness and mental clarity.

EMFs & Headaches

Headaches or violent migraines are one of the top complaints in people who claim and appear to be electro-hypersensitive (EHS).

As I've explained before, EMFs seem to deplete your red blood cells of their oxygen, and give you the same side effects you'd get from hiking in a very high-altitude, low-oxygen environment (called "altitude sickness").

Several research papers have confirmed this effect:

- A study published in 2012 identified that both red and white blood cells, as well as platelets are broken after exposure to cell phone radiation. They also identified that there is an

---

203 As reported by EMF activist Olga Sheean. See emfsafetynetwork.org/wp-content/uploads/2009/09/Personality-changes-caused-by-mobile-telecommunications.pdf
204 emfacts.com
205 sciencedirect.com
206 As reported by Dr. Elizabeth Plourde in *EMF Freedom*. See nature.com/nature/journal/v489/n7416/full/nature11356.html
207 As reported by Dr. Martin Blank in *Overpowered*. See aje.oxfordjournals.org/content/146/12/1037.short
208 Idem. express.co.uk and journals.lww.com

accompanying change in the fluidity of the blood.[209]

- A 2015 article identifies that platelets are subject to oxidative stress and decrease in their oxygen metabolism upon their exposure to LCD monitors.[210]
- When RBCs are exposed to a 900 MHz signal, researcher found that their shape and size changes significantly.[211]

EMFs & Your Eyes

Around 90% of Chinese, Japanese and South Koreans adults suffer shortsightedness — and the exact same trend can be seen in children.[212] Some researchers claim that's because "they work too much"[213] (seriously?), but it might also be because up to 25% of children have been officially recognized as addicted to their smartphone...[214]

The truth is that radar radiation (which uses the same frequency range as cell phones some of the time) has been shown to increase risks of cataracts in otherwise young and healthy military men since the 1950s.[215]

The effects of EMFs on your eyes might be even worse if you wear glasses with metal frames, which act as an antenna and can concentrate the signal coming off your cell phone.[216]

EMFs & Your Ears

In Chapter 3, I made the important (and obviously very serious) recommendation that if you want to follow the current SAR safety standards while using your smartphone, it is recommended not to have ears.

What happens when you ignore this super important warning? Your ears get exposed large amounts of RF radiation — inside and out — including the 3 smallest bones in the human body which are responsible for your hearing.

In a recent interview, researcher Prof. Girish Kumar reported that auditory problem specialists in

209 As reported by Dr. Elizabeth Plourde in *EMF Freedom*. See ncbi.nlm.nih.gov/labs/articles/23054912/
210 Idem. See ncbi.nlm.nih.gov/pmc/articles/PMC4697066/
211 Idem. See ncbi.nlm.nih.gov/pubmed/22676049
212 healthland.time.com
213 huffingtonpost.co.uk
214 bbc.com
215 dtic.mil
216 As reported by Dr. Elizabeth Plourde in *EMF Freedom*. See ncbi.nlm.nih.gov/pubmed/18003202

India are facing an epidemic of hearing problems not in the elderly... in teenagers, and on the exact ear they use to talk on their smartphone all day.[217]

Also, the link between RF radiation and "hearing noises" (including tinnitus, or ringing in the ears) has been known for decades. There's even a term for it — the "Frey" effect[218] — as it was discovered by biologist Allan Frey while he was studying the effects of radars on military men.

EMFs & Your Nervous System

Martin Blank, PhD, cites a series of 3 papers published between 2001 and 2006[219] clearly demonstrating that exposure on one side of the brain slows reaction time of the hand that side governs, and the same is true with exposure on the other side.:

A 2014 review by Redmayne and Johansson[220] confirmed this link and showed that EMFs can damage myelin sheaths — the protective fatty layer which protects your nerves — throughout your body.

This might explain why some electro-hypersensitive people claim they are being affected on a very physical level by EMFs. When surveying residents of Maine after a smart meter got installed at their home, more than 25% of them said they experienced "involuntary muscle contractions".[221]

One study even concluded that sensitive people exposed to the EMFs emitted from a cell phone tower 30 km away from a road are affected so much they could be a problem for traffic safety.[222]

There are also very strong reasons to think EMFs might be a contributing factor in ALS (Lou Gehrig's disease)[223] and MS (multiple sclerosis).[224]

EMFs & Neurodegenerative Diseases

With everything I've shared so far, it's kind of obvious that some researchers have linked EMFs to

---

217 Discussion between Lloyd Burrell and Girish Kumar, PhD, from the Indian Institute of Technology Bombay, as part of ElectricSense.com's EMF Experts Solutions Club. More details at electricsense.com/

218 en.wikipedia.org

219 As reported by Dr. Martin Blank in *Overpowered*. See one of these 3 studies here: ncbi.nlm.nih.gov/pubmed/19194860

220 ncbi.nlm.nih.gov/pubmed/25205214

221 mainecoalitiontostopsmartmeters.org

222 As reported by Dr. Elizabeth Plourde in *EMF Freedom*. See ncbi.nlm.nih.gov/pubmed/21616774

223 Milham, S., MD. (2012). *Dirty Electricity: Electrification and the Diseases of Civilization*. iUniverse

224 As reported by Dr. Elizabeth Plourde in *EMF Freedom*. See ncbi.nlm.nih.gov/pubmed/16687046

Alzheimer's disease and other neurodegenerative conditions (MS falls in that category too), and for a lot of reasons:

- Alzheimer's sufferers have been found to have 33% less GABA than healthy subjects[225] — and EMFs deplete your GABA levels
- Some researchers think that Alzheimer's might be caused by excess calcium in the brain[226] — and EMFs cause excess calcium

Again, this link has been seen for various types of EMF exposure. For example, Swiss researchers have found that the closer you live to high-voltage power lines (which cause high levels of Magnetic Fields) — the more likely you are to develop Alzheimer's.[227]

Alzheimer's Risk Increase For People Who Live Near Power Lines (<50m)[228]

Duration Of Exposure	Increase In Risk
1 year	24%
5 years	50%
10 years	100%

225 Idem. See ncbi.nlm.nih.gov/pubmed/23354600
226 npr.org
227 reuters.com
228 As reported by Dr. Martin Blank in *Overpowered*. See academic.oup.com/aje/article/169/2/167/95445/Residence-Near-Power-Lines-and-Mortality-From

Warning #6: EMFs Might Make You Fat(ter)

Can EMFs Affect Your Weight?[229]
Studies
RF Radiation (V/m)
Effects
A
0.04 - 0.9
↑ Cortisol
B
0.15-0.19
↑ Cortisol, Stress, Adrenaline
C
8.68
↑ Cortisol
D
43.41
↓ Insulin
FCC Limit
61.4
FCC Limit

Can EMFs Affect Your Weight? (Exposure Type)[230]

Type of Exposure	Effect	Study
50-min cell phone call	50-minute cell phone exposure was associated with increased brain glucose metabolism in the region closest to the antenna.	Volkow et al., 2011
One 30-min cell phone call per day for 80 days	Increase blood glucose levels in rats.	Celikozlu et al., 2012
High levels of dirty electricity (>2,000 GS units)	Plasma glucose levels, in the Type 1 and Type 2 diabetic cases reported, respond to electromagnetic pollution in the form of radio frequencies in the kHz range associated with indoor wiring (dirty electricity).	Havas, 2008
High levels of dirty electricity (>2,000 GS units)	Reduced blood sugar levels after Dirty Electricity filters were installed.	Sogabe, 2006
Magnetic fields above 6 mG	Increased blood glucose levels.	Litovitz et al., 1994

I think you're starting to see how everything is interconnected here. EMFs prevent your body from healing — so you get fewer benefits from exercise. EMFs might mess up your mood, killing your motivation to eat well. Who knows... EMFs might even increase your food cravings!

All these things contribute to a reduction in your overall health, making it harder for you to keep a healthy weight.

229 List of detailed references available in Annex 7.
230 List of detailed references available in Annex 8.

EMFs & Blood Sugar

An important factor in keeping a healthy weight is how well you control your blood sugar — and EMFs are happily messing up your ability to keep it stable.

A 2008 paper by Magda Havas has shown that high levels of Dirty Electricity (DE) make it harder for diabetics to control their blood sugar.[231] The unfortunate irony is that most hospitals use fluorescent lights and have very high levels of DE — on top of a few cell phone antennas on the roof, why not?

When it comes to cell phones, conflicting studies show they can either increase your brain's demand in glucose[232] or reduce it.[233]

Research by Paul Héroux, PhD, of the McGill University in Montreal, Canada is pushing it even farther. According to Héroux, EMFs change the setpoint of your metabolism, which has a direct impact on your risks of diabetes and your nervous system.[234]

What this all means in plain English: your cell phone might be swinging your blood sugar up and down, without any of the sensory magic you'd get from munching on a Krispy Creme donut.

EMFs & Stress

The link is obvious. EMFs increase your cortisol, spike your adrenaline, screw up your hormones and make you more prone to anxiety — all of which we can put under the umbrella of "stress".

High cortisol levels are highly correlated with the size of your waist,[235] so reducing your EMF exposure could technically help you keep a healthy weight.

As Elizabeth Plourde reports, there's also a link between EMF exposure and eating disorders like anorexia:[236]

"In a study published in 2013, Dr. Nicole Barbarich-Marsteller in association with other researchers stated it is critical to understand the biochemistry behind anorexia. On investigating rats, they

---

231 ncbi.nlm.nih.gov/pmc/articles/PMC2557071
232 ncbi.nlm.nih.gov/pmc/articles/PMC3184892 and ncbi.nlm.nih.gov/pubmed/22676902
233 ncbi.nlm.nih.gov/pubmed/21915135
234 Discussion between Lloyd Burrell and Paul Héroux, PhD,as part of ElectricSense.com's EMF Experts Solutions Club. More details at http://electricsense.com/. See Héroux's research here: microwavenews.com/news-center/unified-theory-magnetic-field-action
235 unm.edu
236 As reported by Dr. Elizabeth Plourde in *EMF Freedom*. See ncbi.nlm.nih.gov/pmc/articles/PMC3930623/

found that anorexia type behavior is associated with a profound reduction in cells developing in the hippocampus region of the brain.

Since EMFs reduce the number of cells in the hippocampus, as well as reduce GABA functioning, then anorexia behavior is another possible outcome of excess exposure to EMF radiation."

Warning #7: EMFs Might Harm Your Heart

Can EMFs Affect Your Heart? (RF)[237]

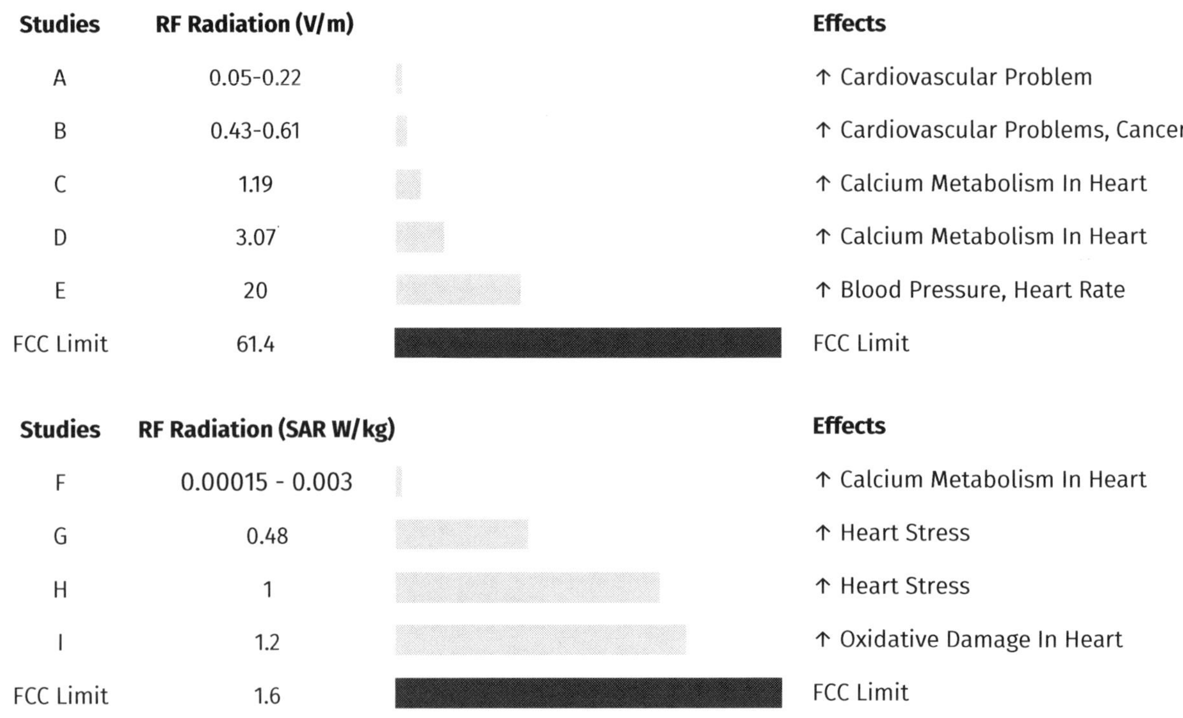

Studies
RF Radiation (V/m)
Effects
A
0.05-0.22
↑ Cardiovascular Problem
B
0.43-0.61
↑ Cardiovascular Problems, Cancer
C
1.19
↑ Calcium Metabolism In Heart
D
3.07
↑ Calcium Metabolism In Heart
E
20
↑ Blood Pressure, Heart Rate
FCC Limit
61.4
FCC Limit
Studies
RF Radiation (SAR W/kg)
Effects
F
0.00015 - 0.003
↑ Calcium Metabolism In Heart
G
0.48
↑ Heart Stress
H
1
↑ Heart Stress
I
1.2
↑ Oxidative Damage In Heart
FCC Limit
1.6
FCC Limit

Can EMFs Affect Your Heart? (MF)[238]

Studies	MF Radiation (mG)	Effects
J	0.00034	↑ Heart Rate
K	24	↓ Antioxidants In Heart
L	42	↑ Heart Stress
M	373	↑ Blood Pressure
N	800	↑ Blood Pressure
ICNIRP Limit[239]	2000	ICNIRP Limit

237 List of detailed references available in Annex 9.
238 List of detailed references available in Annex 10.
239 This is not a typo. The ICNIRP limit for MF occupational exposure is 2,000 mG.

Why does the FDA warn people with pacemakers (artificial hearts) to keep it far away from their cell phone?[240] Because RF radiation messes with the electrical pulses which keep them alive.

Guess what? Non-artificial, human hearts run on electricity too![241] That's probably why "Soviet scientists recognized that EMFs at frequencies between 30 MHz and 300 GHz could affect the human circulatory system (altering heart rate and blood pressure) and nervous system, even at levels too weak to produce thermal effects."[242]

EMFs & Your Blood Pressure: The Lancet has shown that talking on a cell phone can increase your blood pressure by 5 to 10mm.[243]

EMFs & Heart Failure: Martin Pall's research proposes that excess calcium in cells (caused by a disruption of your "VGCCs", the cellular calcium gates) and oxidative stress might be the central cause of heart failure.[244]

EMFs & Reduced HRV: Talking on a cell phone for 20 minutes has decreased the heart rate variability of 32 healthy students, and this effect lasted for 20 minutes following the call. Research by Magda Havas has found the same effect in people exposed to RF radiation coming off "DECT" household cordless phones.[245]

EMFs & Arterial Plaque: Considering that arterial plaque is partially made out of excess calcium[246] and that the heart contains a large density of certain types of VGCCs[247] known to be disrupted by EMFs[248]... there might also be a link here.

EMFs & Inflammation: That's still up for debate, but heart disease is now thought to be an inflammatory disease.[249] Research by Dr. Klinghardt has shown an increase in multiple biomarkers of inflammation (TGF-Beta 1, MMP-9 and copper, which shows chronic inflammation, hormone disruption and neurotransmitter disruption) in people who live in a high EMF environment.[250]

See pse.com/safety/ElectricSafety/Pages/Electromagnetic-Fields.aspx

240 fda.gov

241 webmd.com

242 Blank, M., PhD. (2015). *Overpowered: The Dangers of Electromagnetic Radiation (EMF) and What You Can Do about It.* Seven Stories Press.

243 thelancet.com

244 ncbi.nlm.nih.gov/pmc/articles/PMC3856065

245 magdahavas.com

246 heart.org

247 ucl.ac.uk

248 researchgate.net

249 docsopinion.com

250 Olga Sheean. See Dr. Klinghardt's presentation at this link: youtube.com/watch?v=PktaaxPl7RI&feature=youtu.be

Warning #8: EMFs Might Increase Your Toxic Load

There you go, Nick suddenly went "full tinfoil" and starts to talk about detox, toxins, and toxic load.

While all those words are definitely used to sell a lot of snake oil remedies, the fact remains that our bodies are exposed to many more harmful external toxins that affect our health negatively than our grandparents were. This is what I personally mean by "toxic load".

To understand toxic load, I love the analogy of a bucket. When you're born, your bucket contains some toxins that were given to you by your mother. (Thanks, mom!) In some studies, this bucket has been shown to already contain up to 200 man-made chemicals.[251]

Then, throughout your life, you get exposed to a bunch of toxins in the air you breathe, the food you eat and the water you drink — which gradually fills up this bucket.

Your body is a powerful detoxifying machine though, and it's important to remember that it naturally "detoxes" 24/7 — even when you don't take 15 different overpriced medicinal herbs you bought at Wholefoods.

That being said, in a lot of situations the human body seems to struggle to get rid of certain things like heavy metals — showed to accumulate in your bones[252] — or persistent chemicals like DDT and dioxins[253] — which tend to accumulate faster than the speed at which your liver is able to get rid of them.

There are many ways EMFs might be contributing to making your bucket fuller, faster — until it overflows and becomes an overwhelming burden to your body.

EMFs & Your Detoxification Organs

The first way EMFs might increase your toxic load is by having a direct effect on your main detoxification organs.

Liver: As reported in *Radiation Nation*, one "Chinese study published in May 2014 found that 900 MHz cell phone emissions could cause liver damage in rats by affecting the expression of the Nrf2

251 scientificamerican.com
252 ncbi.nlm.nih.gov/pmc/articles/PMC3047683
253 epa.gov

(a protein that regulates the expression of antioxidant proteins) and inducing oxidative injury.[254]

Kidneys: Pregnant rats exposed to 900 MHz, 1800 MHz, and 2.45 GHz Wifi and mobile phone frequencies for 60 minutes per day gave birth to offsprings with markers of kidney injury.[255]

Bladder: A 2014 study exposing rats to EMF radiation for 8 hours a day found evidence of severe bladder inflammation and tissue damage.[256]

Skin: Again, from *Radiation Nation*: Several studies have found that heat and radiation exposure from laptops can lead to erythema ab igne, otherwise known as toasted skin syndrome, a permanent reddish-brown hyperpigmentation on the surface of the skin.[257]

EMFs have also been linked to histamine reactions on the skin (rashes, tingling, etc.) — similar to the reactions some people have when eating a food they're allergic to.[258]

Can EMFs Affect Your Detox?[259]

Studies	RF Radiation (SAR W/kg)	Effects
A	0.14	↑ Antibodies In Spleen
B	0.38	↑ Oxidative Damage In Liver
C	0.6	↑ DNA Damage In Kidneys And Liver
D	0.88	↑ Oxidative Damage In Liver
E	1.2	↑ Oxidative Damage In Liver
F	1.2	↑ Oxidative Damage In Kidneys
G	1.52	↑ Oxidative Damage In Bladder
H	1.6	↑ Oxidative Damage In Liver
FCC Limit	1.6	FCC Limit

254 As reported by Daniel and Ryan DeBaun in *Radiation Nation*. See ncbi.nlm.nih.gov/pubmed/24941847
255 As reported by Elizabeth Plourde in *EMF Freedom*. See emf-portal.org/en/article/23656
256 Idem. See brazjurol.com.br/july_august_2014/Koca_520_525.pdf
257 As reported by Daniel and Ryan DeBaun in *Radiation Nation*. See ncbi.nlm.nih.gov/pubmed/22031654
258 ncbi.nlm.nih.gov/pubmed/10859662
259 List of detailed references available in Annex 11.

EMFs Let The Bad Stuff In

There are several other ways that EMFs might be increasing your toxic load directly or indirectly:

1. By opening up your blood-brain barrier (BBB) and other protective barriers in your body, which could allow bad stuff to flow in areas it shouldn't, and beneficial substances to leach out

2. By increasing the amount of mercury leaching from your dental amalgams, which seem to be picking up RF radiation like a freaking antenna[260]

3. By enhancing the harmful effects of well-known carcinogens like formaldehyde, small amounts of gamma radiation or mold toxins (aflatoxin)[261]

260 greenmedinfo.com
261 microwavenews.com

Warning #9: EMFs Might Be Harming Your Gut

There's a reason scientists are calling the trillions of bacteria we have in and out of our gut our "second brain".[262] It's now been shown that without these minuscule critters, we'd basically be dead.

After reading this guide and hearing the recommendations I'll make in Chapter 7, chances are you'll think twice about putting a cell phone right next to your ear again — which I personally never do.

But here's some food for thought... if EMF radiation can cause all these problems around your head area, what do you think it does if you replace "head" with "gut" — while you're texting, Instagramming and just playing around with your 4G phone all day 2 inches away from your stomach and intestines? Yeah.

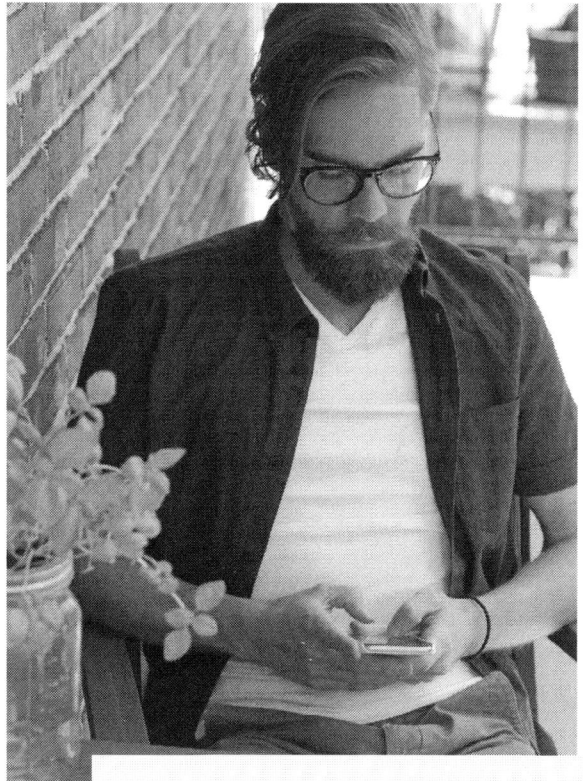

"No worries guys, I'm not exposing my head to RF radiation!"

EMFs & Your Good Bacteria

One of the marks of a healthy gut is a proper ratio between "good" (around 85%) and "bad" (around 15%) bacteria.[263] EMFs have been shown to slow down the growth rate of beneficial bacteria.[264]

Scientists are just starting to discover that bacteria communicate using very low levels of EMFs,[265] so it's unclear how exposing them to an entire EMF soup the way we do could harm them or reduce their health.

And why should you care about the little bugs inside your gut? Among other things, they are responsible for producing at least 90% of your serotonin ("feel-good" hormone)[266], keeping the

262 scientificamerican.com
263 This is a gross oversimplification, but for the sake of our argument here it should be sufficient. articles.mercola.com
264 marioninstitute.com
265 J Microbiol Immunol Infect 2003;36:153-160
266 caltech.edu

bad bacteria under control,[267] neutralizing harmful chemicals like BPA[268] and producing vitamin K.[269]

EMFs & Invaders

EMFs kind of give you a double punch in the gut (pun intended) — by both weakening your good bacteria, and making potential invaders like viruses and parasites way stronger.

In 1997, one surprising study showed that exposure to a 50 Hz Magnetic Field (from household wiring in Europe) activated an otherwise dormant Epstein Barr virus.[270]

Research by Dr. Dietrich Klinghardt has shown that candida and mold cultures can start spewing up to 600 times more biotoxins when exposed to EMF radiation.[271] It seems that these microscopic invaders feel threatened by the invisible signals, and start producing as much poison as they can in order to protect themselves from what probably looks to them like a scary ghost straight out of Scooby-Doo.

I could find two other studies where yeast strains seem to grow faster, stronger and potentially more harmful when exposed to EMFs.[272] Oh, and there's also this shocking 2017 study by Taheri et al. which showed that dangerous bacteria like E. coli and listeria became antibiotic-resistant when exposed to cell phone and wifi signals.[273]

Is that why I keep hearing the top alternative medicine doctors in the world claiming there's an epidemic of mold toxin poisoning, candida issues and other parasitic infections?

EMFs & Autoimmune Diseases

If EMFs have been clearly shown to make the blood-brain barrier (BBB) leak neurotransmitters and let the bad stuff in, there's a strong chance it might be doing the same to your gut — which is usually protected by a very thin layer of cells that's just permeable enough to let nutrients into your blood, without letting larger particles like proteins pass through.

---

267 ncbi.nlm.nih.gov/pmc/articles/PMC4528021
268 greenmedinfo.com
269 bodyecology.com
270 ncbi.nlm.nih.gov/pubmed/9276003
271 it-takes-time.com
272 ncbi.nlm.nih.gov/pubmed/15456218 and ncbi.nlm.nih.gov/pubmed/12452574
273 ncbi.nlm.nih.gov/pubmed/28203122

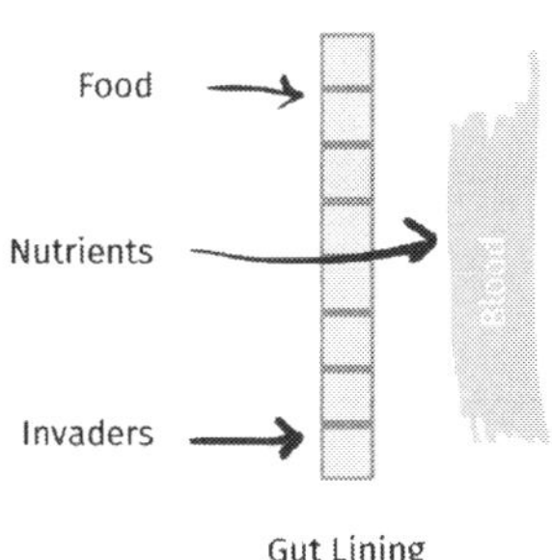

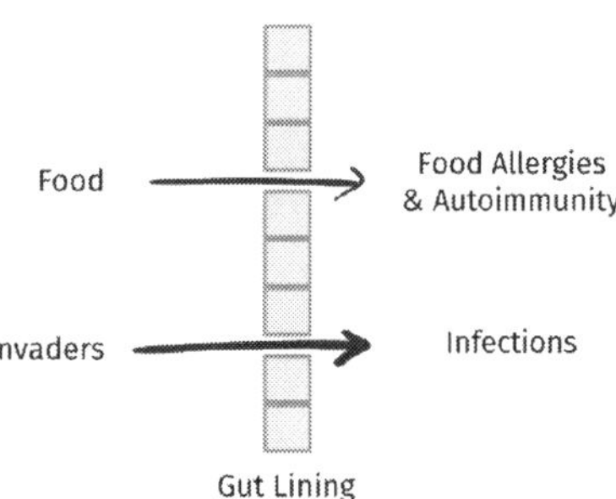

Even if there seems to be a grand total of zero studies on the subject, some thought leaders in the health world like Dr. Jack Kruse are convinced that EMFs are one of the main causes of intestinal permeability, AKA "leaky gut".[274]

If this ends up being true, this means that EMFs might be one of the many reasons that we're seeing an explosion in food allergies and autoimmune diseases such as Celiac, Crohn's, Lupus, Hashimoto's, Rheumatoid Arthritis — all of which can be triggered or worsened by having a leaky gut.[275]

EMFs & Lyme Disease

I might be pushing the envelope here, but what the heck. This is *my* guide after all, and I've been writing for 40 hours in the last 4 days alone. My back hurts.

I think (personal opinion here, based on discussions I've been having with functional medicine practitioners and health enthusiasts) that EMFs might be linked to the massive increase we're seeing in Lyme disease in the US[276] and throughout Europe.[277]

Are EMFs making us more likely to get infected by Lyme? Do EMFs make the Lyme bacteria stronger and more dangerous, or are EMFs getting a bunch of people symptoms similar to those of Lyme disease? I really can't tell at this point — but this link does merit further investigation.

274 jackkruse.com
275 According to Dr. Tom O'Bryan, one of the pioneers of reversing autoimmune diseases. See his book: amazon.ca/dp/B01COAID48/ref=dp-kindle-redirect?_encoding=UTF8&btkr=1
276 npr.org
277 ecdc.europa.eu

Warning #10: EMFs Might Be Harming Your Children

Can EMFs Affect Your Children? (RF)[278]

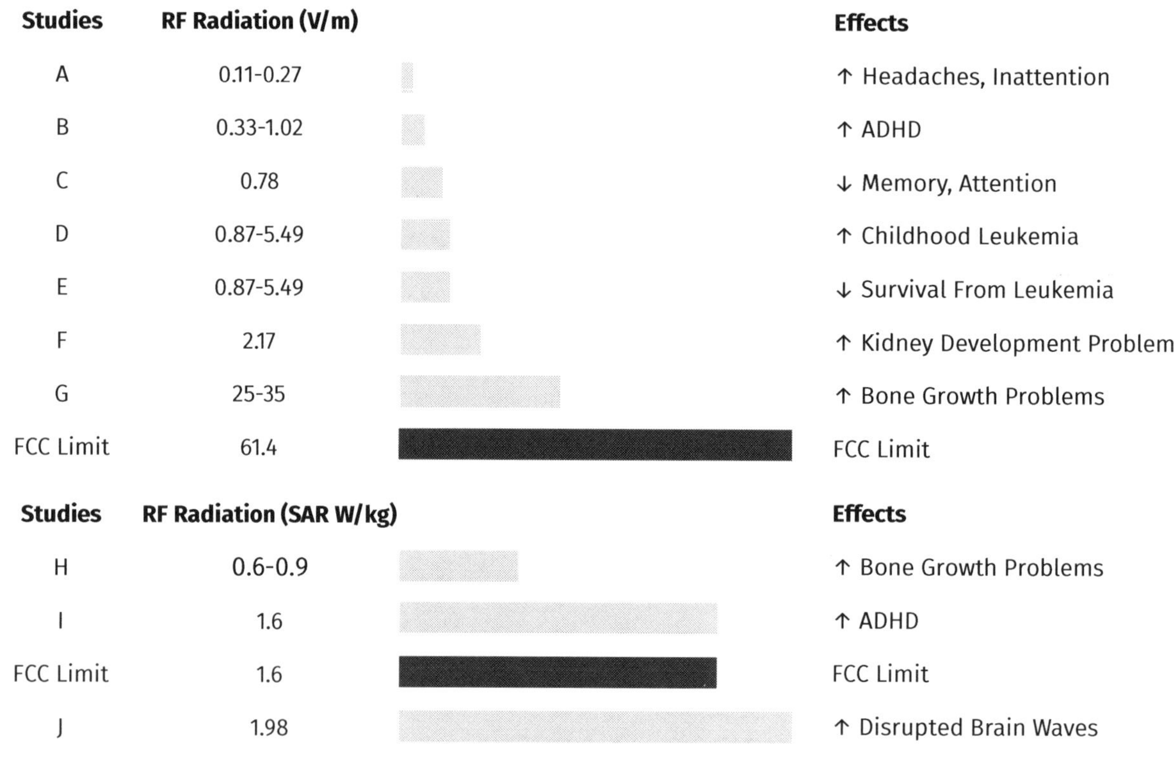

Studies
RF Radiation (V/m)
Effects
A
0.11-0.27
↑ Headaches, Inattention
B
0.33-1.02
↑ ADHD
C
0.78
↓ Memory, Attention
D
0.87-5.49
↑ Childhood Leukemia
E
0.87-5.49
↓ Survival From Leukemia
F
2.17
↑ Kidney Development Problems
G
25-35
↑ Bone Growth Problems
FCC Limit
61.4
FCC Limit
Studies
RF Radiation (SAR W/kg)
Effects
H
0.6-0.9
↑ Bone Growth Problems
I
1.6
↑ ADHD
FCC Limit
1.6
FCC Limit
J
1.98
↑ Disrupted Brain Waves

Can EMFs Affect Your Children? (MF)[279]

Studies	MF Radiation (mG)	Effects
K	2	↑ Risks Of Leukemia
L	2	↑ Risks Of Leukemia
M	4	↑ Risks Of 3 Childhood Cancers
N	10	↑ Heart Development Problems
O	15	↑ Risks Of Obesity
P	30	↑ Heart Development Problems
ICNIRP Limit	2000	ICNIRP Limit

278 List of detailed references available in Annex 12.
279 List of detailed references available in Annex 13.

Can EMFs Affect Your Children? (Other Studies)[280]

Findings	Study
Combined exposure to environmental lead and mobile phone increases risks of ADHD.	Byun et al., 2013
Associations between cell phone use and behavioral problems in young children.	Divan et al., 2012
Children's skulls absorb way more radiation than those of adults.	Gandhi, O. P., 2015
10 year-old children absorb 153% more radiation than adults.	Gandhi, O. P. et al., 2012
Children 11-15 years old using cell phones have an increased risk for headaches, migraines and skin itches.	Chiu et al., 2015
Cell phone use in teenagers increased behavioral problems.	Thomas et al., 2010
Cell phone use increases risks of brain tumors, even at low exposures.	Söderqvist et al., 2011
Positive relationship between cell phone use in children and increased risk or brain tumors.	Morgan et al., 2012
The relationship between MF and childhood leukemia remains consistent with possible carcinogenicity in humans.	Schuz et al., 2016
500% increase in brain cancer risk for teenagers using cell phones before age 20.	Hardell and Carlberg, 2013

I'll get some heavy flak for this one — because everyone gets emotional and angry when there are discussions around what harms or heals children. What the heck, I'm not here to show how Canadian I am, but to tell you the truth like it is.

Everything I've told you about so far applies to children too, but in a scary exponential way — because their bodies absorb up to "60 percent more energy per pound of body weight than an adult. A one-year-old's body can absorb around double the amount."[281]

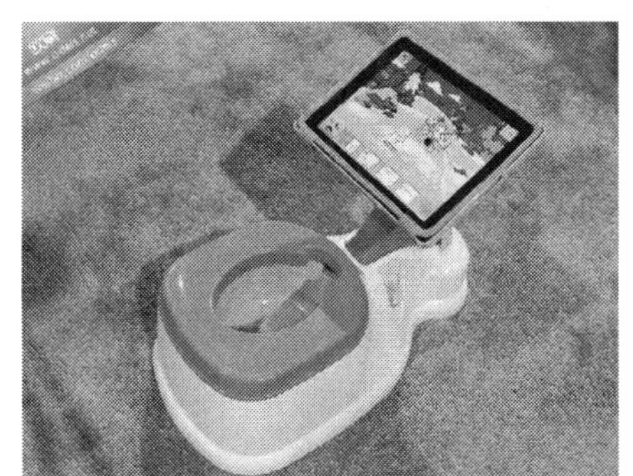

As EMF expert Daniel DeBaun explains, "this is most likely due to the higher water content in children's tissues than adults".[282] You can see why giving a cell phone to a child with

280 List of detailed references available in Annex 14.
281 As reported by Daniel and Ryan DeBaun in *Radiation Nation*. See https://webarchive.nationalarchives.gov.uk/20100910163012/http://www.iegmp.org.uk/documents/iegmp_6.pdf
282 As reported by Daniel and Ryan DeBaun in *Radiation Nation*.

a developing brain is a very bad idea, and why you probably don't want to buy your kid the iPotty for Christmas...

EMFs & Pregnancy

Back in the summer of 1987 when I was still a fetus, I enjoyed a pretty EMF-free environment where I could just swim around, do my thing and grow healthy cells. These days the portrait has changed.

The first EMF risk women face during pregnancy is an increase in their risk of miscarriage, which has been shown in exposure to Magnetic Fields of more than 16 mG,[283] in certain cases to RF radiation exposure,[284] and when using electric blankets[285] — although research is still very unclear here.

Then, the tiny fetus is at risk of seeing its growth slowed down by EMFs from the environment the mom is exposed to, or even from her own cell phone use near her belly.

In animal studies, EMFs have been linked in all aspects of fetal growth, including:

- Kidney development[286]
- Bone growth[287]
- Vascular system growth[288]

Nothing surprising here. If EMFs affect adults the way a lot of solid research shows they might — they also might affect all aspects of fetal development, including the part where a fetus creates around 250,000 nerve cells per minute throughout the pregnancy.[289]

Ironically, as the pregnancy progresses and the baby gets bigger, his exposure levels go way up as he starts pushing against his mother's belly.

EMFs & Newborns

Unsurprisingly, EMF exposure in the womb might lead to consequences that can show up in newborns.

See dx.doi.org/10.1016/j.pathophys.2013.03.001
283 ncbi.nlm.nih.gov/pubmed/11805581
284 ec.europa.eu and ncbi.nlm.nih.gov/pmc/articles/PMC1469943
285 onlinelibrary.wiley.com
286 ncbi.nlm.nih.gov/pubmed/15042631
287 emf-portal.org
288 emf-portal.org and emf-portal.org
289 ncbi.nlm.nih.gov/books/NBK234146

In animal and human studies, fetuses exposed to EMFs in the womb have been shown to be more likely to suffer from a bunch of ailments.

- An exposure to Magnetic Fields higher than 2.5 mG (pretty low) has been correlated with a doubling in risks of childhood obesity[290]
- For every 1 mG increase in the Magnetic Fields levels expecting moms were exposed to, children became 15% more likely to develop asthma later in life[291]
- There are so many studies linking EMF exposure in the womb and neurological changes in children that I'll have to keep you here for a little longer!

EMFs & ADHD

EMFs open up the blood-brain barrier. Obvious link with reduced neurotransmitters in the brain, and therefore with ADHD.[292]

As Elizabeth Plourde reports: "A study published in 2008 looked at over 13,000 mothers and their children who were measured both prenatally (during pregnancy) and postnatally (after delivery) for exposure to cell phone radiation.

They identified that there was a higher score for overall behavioral problems in the children who were exposed to cell phone use, either during fetal development or postnatally from birth to 7 years-old.

They concluded: 'Exposure to cell phones prenatally and, to a lesser degree, postnatally' was associated with behavioral difficulties such as emotional and hyperactivity problems around the age of school entry."[293]

The exact same results have been found in a different set of 28,000 children who had been exposed to cell phone radiation in the womb and at a young age.[294]

Researchers Sam Milham[295] and Magda Havas[296] have found a strong link between high levels of Dirty Electricity (DE) and behavioral problems in children.

290 microwavesnews.com
291 jamanetwork.com
292 ncbi.nlm.nih.gov/pmc/articles/PMC3970207
293 Idem. See ncbi.nlm.nih.gov/pubmed/18467962
294 Idem. See ncbi.nlm.nih.gov/pubmed/21138897
295 Milham, S., MD. (2012). *Dirty Electricity: Electrification and the Diseases of Civilization*. iUniverse
296 stetzerelectric.com

In one case study, Milham reports that a 4th grade teacher saw immediate changes in her students the instant she filtered out the dirty electricity in her classroom using special filters. The teacher even surprisingly confirmed that "she could change the behavior of the children by removing and reinserting the filters" — in just 30 to 45 minutes.

Are we giving children ADHD by trying to teach them in a room filled with 50 different iPads? A lot of EMF activists like Dr. Andrew Goldsworthy think so.[297] It makes me wonder if EMFs were part of the hidden reasons children became "unteachable" after the L.A. district spent $1.3 billion to purchase 500,000 iPads back in 2013...[298]

EMFs & Autism

Yes, he's going there. I get it — talking about the possible causes or contributing factors to the current autism epidemic is like slapping certain parents in the face.

But trust me, nothing I'll share below is my personal opinion. Everything is based on research by independent scientists who just want to find solutions to make the life of autistic children and their families better.

To address the EMF-autism link, let me talk about 3 people who are at the forefront of this issue:

Dr. Dietrich Klinghardt

Investor and EMF activist Peter Sullivan reports: "In 2001, Dr. Dietrich Klinghardt began to notice a higher rate of autism among the children of parents who worked at Microsoft, which is headquartered near his practice outside of Seattle.

Working with a building biologist, he found dramatically higher levels of wireless radiation in the homes of families with autistic children. Dr. Klinghardt now reduces wireless and other electric fields as part of his autism prevention and recovery program. Parents who follow his strict guidelines often see their children improve and even recover in about six months."

In a 2012 video,[299] Dr. Klinghardt boldly states that the EMF-autism link is so strong that he can accurately predict the risks a pregnant mother faces of having an autistic child just by measuring the levels of EMFs in her sleeping environment.

---

297 emfacts.com
298 wired.com
299 youtube.com

Dr. Martin Pall

This guy is definitely keeping himself busy, even if he is technically "retired". In 2015, he did a presentation at the Autism One Conference — where he clearly demonstrated the link between screwed up VGCCs (remember, excess calcium flowing into your cells?) and autism.[300]

I've personally watched every single talk I could find on YouTube from Dr. Pall, and I can tell you that he's always very conservative when saying that one thing *causes* another thing, unless there's incredibly solid science behind his claims.

With that in mind, he now states that "the autism epidemic is *probably* caused by EMF exposure". Excess calcium in cells lead to an inflammatory overload, impaired neuron formation, blood-brain barrier disruption, and a bunch of other processes that could all contribute to the overload autistic children are affected by.

Dr. Toril Jelter and Cindy Sage

After seeing how incredibly fast autistic children seem to get better in a low-EMF environment, Jelter and Sage developed a special protocol for autistic kids that's often cited in the online autism circles.

Their advice is pretty simple. For at least 12 hours per day (at night), shut down the electrical circuits to the child's bedroom — while turning off any wifi router, baby monitor or "DECT" household cordless phone (all of which emit RF radiation).[301]

The results such simple changes can have in some autistic children are incredible. 80% of the children get better in just 2 weeks.

Nothing I've talked about in this section is the definitive proof that EMFs are the sole *cause* of autism. The jury is still out on that. But the evidence that a low-EMF environment helps most autistic kids get better cannot be ignored, and needs further investigation.

---

300 youtube.com
301 clearlightventures.com

The Truth Is... We Don't Know Jack Sh*t.

I figured I would allow myself at least one swear word out of the thousands of words in this guide. Maybe that's because I'm still a little fired up from writing the chapter about children...

Look, the reality here is that we don't know exactly how EMFs affect us. Science doesn't know. The FCC doesn't know. And cell phone manufacturers certainly don't know the whole picture either, or else they would be crapping their pants.

There are a lot of questions that need further study to be definitely answered, like...

1) Are the effects from EMFs cumulative?

We know that exposure to x-rays and other imaging technologies accumulate, which is why we need to restrict their use as much as possible[302] — and why we stopped blasting people's feet with x-rays just to figure out their shoe size like back in the 50s.[303]

Martin Blank warns that "the effect [from EMFs] is cumulative, across a lifetime of exposures."[304] Should we restrict our use of wifi unless it's medically necessary?

2) How are researchers going to study our current EMF exposure?

By the time a study comes out, we're already two new phone generations down the line. The study is barely valid at that point. How can we really study our exposure if the number of devices we're exposed to keeps increasing exponentially?

3) What are the current levels of EMFs in your own bedroom?

What about a kindergarten? What about a hospital room on the top floor, when there are 20 cell phone antennas on the roof? Without spending hundreds on EMF meters and looking like a tinfoil hatter, there's really no way to tell.

4) What levels of EMFs will you be exposed to in 20 years from now?

Everyone believes non-ionizing radiation from wifi does nothing, so we're all good, right?

---

302 medicalnewstoday.com
303 gizmodo.com
304 Blank, M., PhD. (2015). *Overpowered: The Dangers of Electromagnetic Radiation (EMF) and What You Can Do about It.* Seven Stories Press.

5) What are the possible consequences of blasting the entire planet with 24/7 wifi the way corporations like Google and Facebook want to do it?

Their grand plan is to provide every single human being with a 1 Mbps Internet connection. But at what cost?

6) Should you have the legal right to tell your neighbor to turn off his wifi router at night, if it makes you unable to sleep? Should second-hand EMFs be treated like second-hand smoke?

After all, just a few decades ago it was totally fine to smoke on airplanes, even if it made everyone basically cough black tar after their flight.[305] In 1973, they even made "non-smoking" zones mandatory in airplanes.[306]

7) How can we properly study our EMF'ed population when virtually no one is un-exposed, AKA there's no proper "control group"?

I mean, even the Amish are getting on board![307] Will we be able to find anyone on the planet who has never used a cell phone in just a few years from now?

8) What happens when we mix different frequencies of signals together, different kinds of signal modulations, pulsing rates and harmonics — which can all change how our cells react to EMFs?

It's been shown that erratic, pulsed EMFs (like those coming off your phone) can be more harmful than continuous, smooth signals.[308] According to a top EMF engineer, there "are now about 20 modulation systems in widespread common use, plus about 50 or more specialist ones" — and each one of these ways of encoding EMF signals could change how they affect our cells.[309]

9) Why do I keep asking questions when the point has clearly been made 2 minutes ago?

Sorry about that... I tend to get carried away.

The real question here is... what the heck should you do about EMFs while "science" works on the issue, and before the safety guidelines finally catch up with reality?

---

305 nytimes.com
306 sourcewatch.org
307 lancasteronline.com
308 magdahavas.com
309 As shared on mieuxprevenir.blogspot.ca/2017/02/antenna-sickness-is-everywhere-now.html This is 2016 information from UK radio engineer Alasdair Philips in a personal letter to colleagues. Philips is the genius inventor of the Acoustimeter, a broadband audio microwave detector used to identify ambient RF signals.

Chapter 6

CROSSROADS

Do We Need More Research?

Countries Taking EMF Action

What Are Safe Levels?

My jaw dropped each time I heard EMF engineer Daniel DeBaun share this story on multiple interviews.

Hand on the bible, that's what Joseph Cullman, the former CEO of tobacco industry giant Philip Morris told the press, the judges, and the public when asked if there was a clear link between smoking and lung cancer.

He also gave this nugget of some 1971 wisdom to all expecting moms:[310]

*"It's true that babies born from women who smoke are smaller, but they're just as healthy as babies born from women who do not smoke. And some women would prefer having smaller babies. ***all smiles***"*

I mean, the guy was an OB-GYN — he *must* have known what he was talking about!

The tobacco industry has been so successful in manufacturing doubt in both policy makers, politicians and the public that its practices gave rise to the term "tobacco science" — which refers to science that's manufactured to make an industry profit from the status quo.

Of course, this echoes what the Telecom industry (that's multiple times bigger than Big Pharma, by the way[311]) has been saying for the past 4 decades. "We need more research."

Other authorities like the FDA put it more bluntly. They will not act to protect consumers unless cell phones are definitely proven dangerous.[312] Not their job.

Then there are companies who manufacture tech that they claim emits "safe" amounts of EMF radiation. Unfortunately, it turns out that... it's not their job either!

As bestselling author and biohacker Dave Asprey shares in *Radiation Nation*, he "recently took part in an event with several chief technology officers of some of the world's top virtual reality companies." When he asked who on their incredible team of top-level engineers had the important responsibility to make sure their devices are safe for the human brain, he received the obvious but

310 youtube.com
311 Big Pharma was a global industry of $1.05 trillion in 2016 (fool.com), while the Telecom industry in the US alone is planned to reach $1.3 Trillion before 2020 (finance.yahoo.com)
312 pbs.org

cringing answer... "No one. It's not our job."[313]

Well folks, it sure looks like we're at a crossroads here — and that we have to carefully pick the way to go.

---

313 DeBaun, D. and DeBaun, R. (2017). *Radiation Nation: The Fallout of Modern Technology — Your Complete Guide to EMF Protection & Safety: The Proven Health Risks of Electromagnetic Radiation (EMF) & What to Do Protect Yourself & Family*. Icaro Publishing.

Choice #1: The "Wait Until It's Proven" Approach

"The primary reason for inaction is the meme repeatedly cited by the wireless industry: there is NO CONCLUSIVE PROOF of harm."

- Martin Blank, PhD

You're an adult. You have the full rights to ignore everything you've read so far, and move on with your life. You can even write a clever rant on Facebook about how "unproven" EMF science is, flag this entire issue as "pseudoscience", tell everyone how much of a quack Nicolas Pineault is — and you'd be at least partially right.

This is the "wait until it's proven approach" — where you choose not to think or act by yourself, blindly trusting what the Government and official authorities tell you is safe. Because they'll figure it out. *Eventually.*

Unfortunately, saying this kind of approach has had a "horrible" track record throughout recent history would be a grave understatement...

Issue	Early Warning Signs "Wait, this might be a serious problem!"	Change In Policy "How did we not stop this madness sooner?"	Delay	Known Consequences "Oops!"
Asbestos	1906[314]	Complete ban in 2005 (European Union)	99 years[315]	• Still killing 10,000+ people every year in the US alone

314 asbestos.com
315 europa.eu
316 eionet.kormany.hu
317 worstpolluted.org
318 wired.com

Issue	Early Warning Signs "Wait, this might be a serious problem!"	Change In Policy "How did we not stop this madness sooner?"	Delay	Known Consequences "Oops!"
Lead in gasoline	1925[316]	Complete ban in 1996 (USA)[317]	71 years	• 68 million children with toxic levels of lead[318] • 5,000 annual deaths from lead-induced heart disease • Measurable drop in IQ scores during the leaded gas era • Increased violent crime rates in the 20th century
Trans fats	1957[319]	To be banned in 2018 (USA)[320]	61 years	• 42,174 annual deaths from cardiovascular disease[321] (extrapolated, this would be 2.5M deaths in 60 years)
PCE in tap water	1925	To be banned in 2022 (France)[322]	97 years	• Kidney cancer • Non-Hodgkin lymphoma • Cardiac defects (Numbers unclear, issue still going on today)
Smoking	1949[323, 324]	First bans in public places in 1995 (California)[325]	Still going on today...	• Still killing 1.5-2M people a year from lung cancer alone[326]

319 washingtonpost.com
320 nytimes.com
321 arstechnica.com
322 chemicalwatch.com
323 theguardian.com
324 Although we can find warning signs about the dangers of smoking dating back from 1602: ncbi.nlm.nih.gov/pubmed/15198996
325 en.wikipedia.org
326 tobaccocontrol.bmj.com

And if you thought I just ruined your day with all this doom and gloom stuff, I'm sorry I have to share one more example I read in Elizabeth Plourde's amazing book that shows how human nature tends to screw things up:[327]

"[In the 1840s], Dr. Ignaz Semmelweis identified that doctors going from autopsy to assisting in childbirth were responsible for the 20% of the women who were continually dying from childbed fever (puerperal infection).

He arranged an experiment of washing hands between autopsy and assisting with childbirths. That simple act reduced the outrageously high number of mothers dying down to only 1%.

But, because the bacteria could not be seen, doctors refused to believe they were infecting their patients, and kept on killing 20% of our women for an additional 30 years before washing of hands was adopted as an essential, common sense answer that is necessary to save lives."

Unfortunately for your sanity, the end of the story is even worse... wait for it... "Dr. Semmelweis died in a mental institution before being able to see his life-saving research become accepted as common sense." Ouch.

Am I suggesting that policy makers always screw up, and that everything they claim is safe these days is actually not? Of course not.

What I am saying is that if we learned anything from these past mistakes, we should listen to the early warning signs — for example, thousands of studies that show low-level EMFs might be harmful — and then act with precaution.

327 Plourde, E., PhD, and Plourde, M., PhD. (2016). *EMF Freedom — Solutions for the 21st Century Pollution* - 3rd Edition. New Voice Publications.

Instead of doing just that, we're exponentially increasing the amount of EMFs we're all exposed to, we're right about to upgrade all networks to 5G which means multiplying the number of cell phone antennas we use tremendously, we're connecting 50 billion new devices by 2020[328] thanks to the "Internet Of Things" and we're even planning to blast a constant EMF signal to every plant, animal and living thing on the entire planet using satellites or freaking giant balloons.

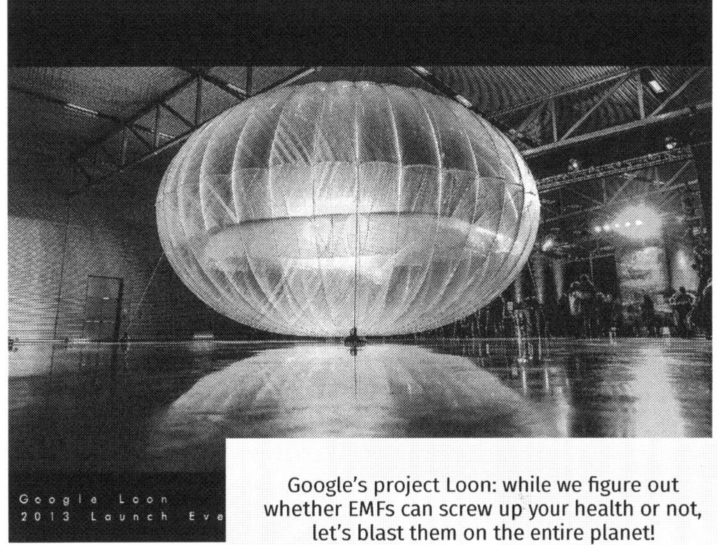

Google's project Loon: while we figure out whether EMFs can screw up your health or not, let's blast them on the entire planet!

May I innocently suggest none of these sounds like being "cautious"?

328 singularityhub.com

Choice #2: The Precautionary Principle

The Precautionary Principle instructs us that in the face of serious threats, a lack of scientific certainty never justifies inaction.

- Yes, Martin Blank, PhD, once again. Can't get enough of this guy.[329]

Remember when I told you that believing that "Science" has everything figured out is like believing in Santa?

The same goes for people who still think that if you can purchase a cell phone, it means it's inherently safe — because the Government and regulatory agencies have your back, and always rely on the precautionary principle. But as you can already guess, it's a philosophy that's in fact very rarely applied in our money-driven society.

pre·cau·tion·ar·y prin·ci·ple

noun

the principle that the introduction of a new product or process whose ultimate effects are disputed or unknown should be resisted. It has mainly been used to prohibit the importation of genetically modified organisms and food.

I would explain what the precautionary principle is to the average Joe on the street using two words: common sense.

Following this principle, even if there were just one study, one warning sign that maybe the EMFs we're constantly bathing in *might* be harmful in the long run... we should probably force manufacturers to create safer devices that emit less EMFs, right? Just in case!

Of course, you need to give these manufacturers time to change their ways. It'll likely cost them billions to create safer products, and we don't want to crash the economy, do we?

329 Blank, M., PhD. (2015). *Overpowered: The Dangers of Electromagnetic Radiation (EMF) and What You Can Do about It*. Seven Stories Press.

But still, using the precautionary principle is all about putting human health before profits, and most of all — learning from our past mistakes that clearly show that humanity has this uncanny ability to screw up its environment, and then feel sorry it has to clean up its mess afterwards.

This is not just the opinion of Nicolas Pineault, an almost-famous health journalist who works in his PJs on most days — but the opinion of thousands of independent organizations, scientists, doctors, thinkers and people who have no intention to let us repeat the same mistakes we did with cigarette smoke, asbestos, lead, trans fats and so many other issues.

Since 2002, many groups of scientists and concerned citizens have been joining forces to command urgent changes in our EMF policies and safety guidelines worldwide.[330]

Resolution/Group	Country	# Of Scientists & Doctors	Year	Conclusion
Salzburg Resolution[331]	Austria	19	2002	A limit value of 0.1 μW/cm2 (0.2 V/m) is recommended. That's 10,000X less than current FCC safety limits.
Freiburger Appeal[332]	Germany	52 authors, signed by 1000 doctors	2002	Current mobile communications technology are among the fundamental triggers of disease.
Irish Doctors' Environmental Association (IDEA)[333]	Ireland	N/A	2005	The Irish Government should urgently research into the adverse health effects of exposure to all forms of non-ionizing radiation.
Seletun Statement[334]	Norway	5	2001	It has become obvious that new, biologically-based public exposure standards taking into account non-thermal exposures are urgently needed to protect public health.
Bioinitiative Report[335]	USA	36	2007 and 2012	New safety limits must be established. Health agencies should act now.

330 semanticscholar.org
331 magdahavas.com
332 magdahavas.com
333 emrpolicy.org
334 magdahavas.com
335 bioinitiative.org
336 magdahavas.com
337 emfscientist.org
338 ncbi.nlm.nih.gov/pubmed/27454111

Resolution/Group	Country	# Of Scientists & Doctors	Year	Conclusion
International Doctors Appeal[336]	Germany	N/A	2012	Follow-up to the Freiburg Appeal of 2002. Calls for stricter guidelines and more urgent action.
International Electromagnetic Field Scientist Appeal[337]	USA	5 authors, signed by 225 scientists	2015	The agencies setting safety standards have failed to impose sufficient guidelines to protect the general public, particularly children who are more vulnerable to the effects of EMFs.
The European Academy for Environmental Medicine Guidelines[338]	European Union	15	2016	Recommends very strict guidelines. For example, an exposure to wifi at night of just 0.02 V/m — 100,000 times less than current FCC safety limits.
The Non-Tinfoil Guide To EMFs	Canada	Zero. Just a regular guy trying to figure things out.	2017	"Uh-oh. I think we might be in trouble."

Anti-Technology?

Trust me — none of these scientists want to destroy cell phones, ban wifi routers, and go back to the Stone Age. But they all agree that the way we currently do things isn't right, and that guidelines need to change, like yesterday.

These good folks all agree that the precautionary principle should be applied here — which means we need to act now, not in 40 years when EMFs will finally be deemed totally safe, totally unsafe, or somewhere in the middle.

Applying the precautionary principle isn't some kind of flowery utopia invented by barefoot hippies — it's been applied before in recent history.

The most obvious example is the entire Endangered Species Act (ESA) of 1973,[339] which "provides for the conservation of species that are endangered or threatened throughout all or a significant portion of their range, and the conservation of the ecosystems on which they depend."

In other words, the entire goal of this act is to use the precautionary principle and do something *before* we reach the level of complete scientific proof. As Martin Blank puts it eloquently... "after all, once we have definitive proof that a species is extinct, it's too late to prevent extinction."[340] Duh.

Luckily, the ESA was no one-hit wonder for humanity.

In 1989, chlorofluorocarbons (CFCs) — a kind of plastic that was used in styrofoam cups, aerosols and a bunch of other products — were phased out worldwide, just 14 years after the early warning signs that they might be destroying the planet's fragile ozone layer.

I'll let Kevin Griffin from the Vancouver Sun tell the story, he does it better than me:[341]

"In 1973, chemists Frank Sherwood Rowland and Mario Molina at the University of California, Irvine noticed that something happened as CFCs rose through the atmosphere to the stratosphere. After an estimated 50 to 100 years, ultraviolet radiation starts to break down CFCs and cause the release of a chlorine atom. They theorized that the chlorine would be enough to affect the ozone layer.

Although the scientists' findings were disputed by chemical corporations ***[of course!]****, their findings*

339 nmfs.noaa.gov
340 Blank, M., PhD. (2015). *Overpowered: The Dangers of Electromagnetic Radiation (EMF) and What You Can Do about It*. Seven Stories Press.
341 vancouversun.com

were supported by numerous scientific studies including a significant report by the British Antarctic Survey in 1985. Abnormally low concentrations of ozone near the South Pole, they speculated, were linked to increased CFCs in the atmosphere. This lead to a time-lapse visual representation of the famous 'ozone hole.'

One of the significant milestones occurred on Jan. 1, 1989 when a treaty called the Montreal Protocol ***[French Canadians are just that smart]*** *on Substances that Deplete the Ozone Layer came into effect. The Montreal Protocol, negotiated two years earlier and signed by Canada, was the first international treaty to deal with a global environmental challenge.* ***[120 different countries got together to sign the agreement and start to phase out the use of CFCs]***

The worldwide ban on CFCs happened relatively quickly. It went from a problem identified by scientists to effective action by politicians within 14 years."

This story has the perfect happy ending. The good guys win, the bad guys hopefully get what they deserve, everyone has a good laugh, and you're all smiles as the credits start rolling down.

In 1995, Frank Sherwood Rowland and Mario Molina (along with Paul J. Crutzen) ended up getting a Nobel prize for their work and its impact on saving the ozone layer.

Even better — the US National Oceanic and Atmospheric Administration confirmed in 2006 that the Montreal Protocol led to real change, and that "the total abundance of ozone-depleting gases in the atmosphere has begun to *decrease* in recent years."[342]

Sure, industries around the world had to change their products in a serious way. But did people really notice how different their cheap office coffee tasted when held in a CFC-free styrofoam cup? And did aerosols suddenly stop smelling like white daisies or Amazonian falls?

I may be an optimist — even if I realize this entire guide probably displays the opposite — but I think the same precautionary principle can, and will soon be applied to EMFs as the word finally gets out.

We can create devices with lower emissions, lower power, different signal encoding — and even possibly make them completely "biocompatible" with the human body, removing virtually any harm they could cause.

342 esrl.noaa.gov

Yes, there are good news coming up. Good news that unfortunately we don't hear about much in North American media — which is why most people reading this will be in total shock once they realize how seriously other countries think the EMF issue is.

As I'm writing these lines in May 2017, there are dozens of different countries that have taken action to put stricter EMF safety guidelines in place like removing wifi, cell phone antennas and other EMF-emitting devices from playgrounds, hospitals, schools and other places where children or sick people might suffer more from EMF exposures, and much, much more.

I think these policies not only show how serious the problem is and that concerns about EMFs are definitely not just some tinfoil delusion — but also what real-life solutions we can all implement to protect ourselves, today.

Keep in mind that the list of countries who are implementing safety measures is by no means definitive. It's changing by the minute.

Before moving on, I want to send a special thanks to Daniel & Ryan DeBaun from *Radiation Nation* and the Environmental Health Trust for the massive amount of hours they spent compiling the research about policies around the world. Without their work, none of this would have been possible.

Warning Labels

Warning labels are the first step in consumer awareness — as we've seen happen with cigarettes.

I personally think we should add a label on every cell phone which says "do not keep your cell phone in your pocket or a laptop on your lap if you ever want children", but what other countries are currently doing is at least a good start.

Country	Warning Label[343]	Since
Israel[344]	This mobile phone emits non-ionizing radiation; details and information about the radiation levels of this mobile phone model and the maximum permissible level of radiation are included in the attached leaflet.	2002
Belgium	Think about your health — use your mobile phone moderately, make your calls wearing an earpiece and choose a set with a lower SAR value.	2013
France[345]	Requires SAR to be displayed on the label of all cell phones... for what it's worth.	2015
Canada	Cell phones may be possibly carcinogenic to humans.	2015, bill did not pass[346]
USA — City of Berkeley, CA	Might cause cancer, keep away from children and pregnant women.	2016
USA — States of California,[347] Pennsylvania,[348] Hawaii,[349] Maine,[350] Oregon,[351] Ohio[352] and Massachusetts[353]	Unclear. "The goal is to inform all citizens about possible health dangers that have been linked to microwave radiation."	Bills did not pass

343 ehtrust.org
344 tnuda.org.il
345 lemonde.fr
346 c4st.org
347 cnet.com
348 legis.state.pa.us
349 capitol.hawaii.gov
350 mainelegislature.org
351 wweek.com
352 congress.gov
353 sites.google.com

Cell Phone Antennas

While the FCC is busy pushing the next-generation "5G" networks[354] that are basically going to require the installation of tiny antennas on every street corner[355] and every traffic light pole[356] — a handful of other countries are busy removing antennas from their environment because they consider them a real health hazard. Go figure.

Country	Policy On Antennas	Since
Canada, Vancouver School Board[357]	Cell phone antennas can't be installed within 1,000 feet from school property or childcare facilities.	2005
India, state of Rajasthan[358]	Cell towers are being dismantled by the thousands, being removed from the vicinity of schools, colleges, hospitals and playgrounds because of radiation "hazardous to life."	2012
Chile	Limits the power of antennas. Can't be installed near "sensitive areas" where children, elderly and medically compromised people would be exposed.	2012
France	Citizens can fight against their placement, cities can refuse them. Also, a map of high-emission antennas will be made available to the public.	2015
Greece	Cell phone antennas can't be installed around schools or nurseries.	Unclear
New Zealand[359]	Cell phone antennas can't be installed around schools.	Unclear
Argentina[360]	Mandatory public consultation before installing antennas.	In Progress

As I pointed out in Chapter 2, the US Telecom companies still have immunity (thanks to the 1996 Telecommunications Act) when it comes to the placement of cell phone antennas. In fact, you couldn't even sue them if you had irrefutable scientific proof that living or working close to an antenna gave you cancer.

354 usatoday.com
355 cio.com
356 twincities.com
357 council.vancouver.ca
358 ecfsapi.fcc.gov
359 education.govt.nz
360 nuevocronista.com

Wifi In Schools

The debate is on. On one hand, certain parents feel that the fear of wifi is completely nuts, because they still believe the physicists' fairy tale about how non-ionizing radiation cannot possibly harm the human body.

And on the other hand, you have concerned parents who are taking action, and trying to figure out what happens when you have 40 iPads and multiple wifi routers blasting away in a small room.

There's also the fact that certain children whose desk is right next to or under a wifi router are exposed to EMF radiation levels dozens of times higher than children who are sitting far from it.

In one case, a parent measured levels of 19.41 V/m right under the router[361] — more than what you'd get exposed to by talking on a 4G/LTE cell phone all day, every day.

Country	Policy On Wifi	Since
USA	Multiple organizations like the American Academy of Pediatrics issued recommendations to reduce wireless exposures to children.	2013
Israel[362]	Wireless networks banned in preschools and kindergartens. 1st & 2nd grade Internet is limited to 3h/week. 3rd grade Internet limited to 8h/week.	2013
France	Banned from nursery schools and spaces dedicated to children under 3 years old. Wifi should be "OFF" when not in use.	2015
Italy, Piemonte region[363]	Limiting the use of wifi in schools.	2015
Taiwan	Use of electronic devices such as iPads, televisions and smartphones banned in children under the age of two.	2015

361 parentsforsafetechnology.org

Country	Policy On Wifi	Since
Cyprus[364]	Wifi is banned from kindergartens and wireless deployment halted in elementary schools.	2017
Finland[365]	One primary school installed "OFF" switches for wifi routers, only turning the devices on when needed. Banned from certain preschools and daycare centers.[366]	2017
Spain[367]	Wants to ban wifi from schools.	In Progress

362 cms.education.gov.il
363 cr.piemonte.it
364 ehtrust.org
365 ehtrust.org
366 flanderstoday.eu
367 tercerainformacion.es

Children Using Cell Phones Or Other Wireless Devices

"In a world where a drug cannot be launched without proof that it is safe, where the use of herbs and natural compounds available to all since early Egyptian times are now questioned, their safety subjected to the deepest scrutiny, where a new food cannot be launched without prior approval, the idea that we can introduce Wifi and mobile phones without restrictions around our 5-year-olds is double-standards gone mad."

- Chris Woollams, Editor, Integrated Cancer and Oncology News CEO, CANCERactive[368]

It's obvious. Wireless devices were never meant to be used by children. We know their bodies absorbs more radiation, and that there's no way on Earth they can stay within the already-broken SAR "safety" guidelines.

And yet, manufacturers are coming up with new devices that emit RF radiation and that are directly created for or marketed to children, including:

- The infamous iPotty I told you about in Chapter 5
- Baby monitors that emit RF radiation 24/7, instead of being voice activated (which would emit 99% less) like in Europe[369]
- Bluetooth diapers that ping your phone when it's wet — planning to hit the market in late 2017[370]
- Wearable Bluetooth devices for babies that can track their health in real time, emitting RF radiation close to their body every second of every day[371]

Fortunately, you're not the only one who thinks this is close to pure madness.

368 Moyer, D. (2014). *Beyond Mental Illness: Transform the Labels, Transform a Life.* Xlibris Corp.
369 According to Magda Havas, PhD, from a 2016 talk she gave in Vermont: youtube.com/watch?v=YFhPkK82ntw
370 techcrunch.com
371 wearables.com

Country	Policy On Children & Cell phones	Since
France	At the request of the buyer, equipment reducing cell phone radiation exposures to the head for children less than 14 years should be provided. Cell phone advertising aimed at children younger than 14 is banned.	2010
Canada	Health Canada recommends citizens to "encourage children under the age of 18 to limit their cell phone usage".	2011
Ireland[372]	We may not truly understand the health effects of cell phones for many years. The sensible thing to do is to adopt a precautionary approach rather than wait to have the risks confirmed. Children should be encouraged to use mobile phones for "essential purposes only".	2011
Belgium	Total ban on cell phone advertising aimed at children.	2013

Few countries address this issue right now and the average American child gets his first smartphone at 6 years old...[373] but things will change if the government adopts stricter guidelines on the amount of EMF radiation children are allowed to be exposed to.

372 hse.ie
373 deseretnews.com

Official Recognition Of Electro-Hypersensitivity (EHS)

I barely touched on the politics and philosophical issues of the current EMF mess we're in, and for a good reason — I wanted to keep this guide short, and as easy to digest as possible.

But if you allow me to be dead honest about what's happening to people suffering from electro-hypersensitivity (EHS) around the world, I would say it's a freaking crime against humanity.

If we use the very conservative estimates that 3% of all people exposed to EMFs are so sensitive that they can't even be around a wifi router without experiencing debilitating symptoms... it means that millions and millions of people around the world are suffering — often in silence, guilt and isolation.

I've heard reports of people being so sensitive to EMFs of different kinds that they can instantly sense that someone forgot to put their phone on "airplane mode". Some even get very distinct different symptoms from cell phones, from wifi, from "DECT" household cordless phones, and from cell phone towers — which makes their body a very effective EMF Meter.

Some of them get hives all over their body. Some of them get neurological symptoms so strong they can barely walk for days, or have a hard time speaking. I even heard Michael Neuert — an EMF mitigation specialist from California with more than 30 years of experience — say that one of his clients is so sensitive that she can sense a cell phone signal that's 1,000 feet from her body.

No, it's not in their head — just like suffering from the Celiac disease (a severe gluten allergy which triggers your immune system into attacking your own body) is not psychological.

Celiac sufferers are so sensitive to gluten that eating just 5ppm — that's equivalent to a few breadcrumbs — of it can make them sick,[374] or worse, bedridden for days. Even breathing the delicious smell of fresh bread coming off their local bakery can be debilitating to them.[375]

It's about time that every single country in the world recognizes that EHS is a real handicap, just like the Swedes have done back in 1995.[376]

374 glutenfreetraveller.com
375 glutenfreehomemaker.com
376 eloverkanslig.org

Country	Policy On EHS Sufferers	Since
USA	The American with Disabilities Act (ADA) recognizes EHS.[377]	2002
Canada	EHS is recognized by the Canadian Human Rights Commission.[378]	2007
Australia[379]	A handful of schools will accommodate children that suffer from EHS. Several legal cases of EHS sufferers have been won.[380]	2013
Italy[381]	The Piemonte region has policies to be considerate of EHS people. EHS-safe areas have been created.	2015
France	A woman in France was compensated after the jury recognized she indeed suffered from EHS.[382] EHS-safe areas have been created.	2015
Spain[383]	One city has started implementing a new plan to help sufferers of MCS (multiple chemical sensitivities) or EHS. One legal ruling has recognized that EHS is a serious disability.[384]	2015

377 ecfsapi.fcc.gov
378 aseq-ehaq-en.ca
379 ehtrust.org
380 itnews.com.au
381 cr.piemonte.it
382 thestar.com
383 afectadasporlosrecortessabitarios.wordpress.com
384 beingelectrosensitive.blogspot.ca

Stricter Standards

Volts per meter. Microwatts per square meter. Milligauss. If all this jargon triggers headaches or anxiety symptoms for you — that's normal.

These things will all start making sense in the next chapter, as I'm going to show you exactly *what you can do* to stay within what I — and experts who follow the precautionary principle instead of the status quo — consider a "safe" amount of EMF exposure.

The truth is that no one knows for sure what levels are safe — and that everyone is still trying to figure things out.

Different organizations around the world and different governments have proposed new guidelines that may not be definitive (only the future will tell), but that are definitely safer than the non-existent ones we have in North America. Let's look at them.

Radio Frequency (RF)

Quick Reminder

- **Type of EMF:** Radio Frequency (RF)
- **Also Called:** Microwaves
- **Measured In:** V/m (volts per meter) or uW/m2 (microwatts per square meter)[385]
- **Likes To:** Bounce around 24/7
- **Usual Sources:** Wifi, cell phones, tablets, anything Bluetooth, smart meters, cell antennas, baby monitors, "DECT" household cordless phones, microwave ovens

RF Guidelines Around The World[386,387]

Authority	Safety Limit (V/m)
USA	61.4
Belgium	21
Russia, China	6
Italy, Luxembourg, Switzerland	6
Building Biology	0.06
Bioinitiative Report	0.03
EUROPAEM	0.02
Austria	0.02
Mother Nature	0.00002

RF radiation safety limits vary quite a lot from country to country. One thing is sure... most countries seem to think that the FCC standards are completely wrong. Austria, for example, allows levels 3,070X lower than the FCC allows.[388]

385 Here's why I decided to stick with V/m for any RF measurement: powerwatch.org.uk/science/unitconversion.asp

386 Thanks to emfs.info for the incredible safety limit compilation they published in August 2016. See emfs.info/wp-content/uploads/2015/07/standards-table-August-2016.pdf

387 List of detailed references available in Annex 15.

388 When calculated in Volts/meters, which I use throughout this guide. When calculated in uW/m2

The actual standards are way more complicated than what I'm showing you here, but I decided to simplify things because doing engineer-level math is not the goal of this guide.

Simply understand that the levels of RF radiation which are considered safe might differ depending on the source of EMFs (wifi, Bluetooth or a cell phone), the frequency, pulsing and modulation of the signal, the duration of exposure, and whether this exposure is happening at night or in the middle of the day.

(power density), the FCC allows levels 1,000,000 times higher. Don't worry about these numbers too much — it's complicated stuff reserved for the EMF nerds.

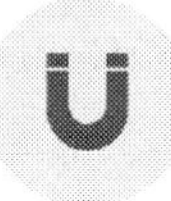

Magnetic Fields (MF)

Quick Reminder

- **Type of EMF:** Magnetic Fields (MF)
- **Measured In:** mG (milligauss)
- **Likes To:** Create a static field which decreases very quickly when you distance yourself from the source
- **Usual Sources:** Breaker panel, faulty household wiring, electric current on water or gas pipes, motors and transformers, high-voltage power lines, solar panels

MF Guidelines Around The World[389,390]

Authority	Safety Limit (mG)
IEEE	9040
ICNIRP	2000
Council of the EU	1000
Argentina	250
Belgium	100
Switzerland	10
Netherlands, Norway	4
Israel	2
Lowest level linked with leukemia	2
EUROPAEM	1
Building Biology	1
Bioinitiative Report	1
Mother Nature	0.000002

389 Thanks to emfs.info for the incredible safety limit compilation they published in August 2016. See emfs.info/wp-content/uploads/2015/07/standards-table-August-2016.pdf

390 List of detailed references available in Annex 16.

Unfortunately, there are thousands of times fewer studies around Magnetic Fields than around cell phones, wifi and other RF-emitting devices. Also, most of the research dates back from the 70s, 80s and 90s — when there were a lot of concerns around the construction of high-voltage power lines and their potential health impacts.

Still, certified Building Biologists and independent researchers like the authors of the 2007 and 2012 Bioinitiative report have formulated clear recommendations about what levels of these fields they think we should be exposed to on an everyday basis — usually based on the lowest level we've seen increase risks of childhood leukemia.

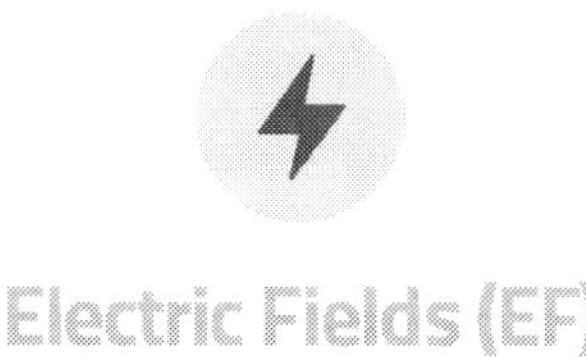

Electric Fields (EF)

Quick Reminder

- **Type of EMF:** Electric Fields (EF)
- **Measured In:** V/m (volts per meter) or mV (millivolts)[391]
- **Likes To:** Electrify your body without you ever noticing
- **Usual Sources:** Standard household wiring, ungrounded 2-prong lamps, most ungrounded electronics, stray current in soils, power strips and other cords

EF Guidelines Around The World[392,393]

Authority	Safety Limit (V/m)
IEEE	10,000
ICNIRP	5000
Council of the EU	5000
Argentina	3000
Costa Rica	2000
Poland	1000
Russia, Slovenia	500
Building Biology	1.5
EUROPAEM	1
Mother Nature	0.0001

International guidelines around Electric Fields (EF) coming off standard electricity in the walls of your home are even more blurry.

391 When using what Building Biologists call the "body voltage method", which uses one of these kits to assess how much voltage from surrounding Electric Fields is actually getting into your body: slt.co/Products/BodyVoltageKits/

392 Thanks to emfs.info for the incredible safety limit compilation they published in August 2016. See emfs.info/wp-content/uploads/2015/07/standards-table-August-2016.pdf

393 List of detailed references available in Annex 17.

Building Biologists like Oram Miller — who helps clients all over the West Coast reduce EMF levels in their homes — say that EF are the most underrated and misunderstood kinds of EMFs people can be exposed to.[394]

It's also well recognized within the Building Biology profession that EF can seriously impair your body's ability to get in that deep, healing stage 4 "REM" sleep, on top of:[395]

- Reducing your normal night time production of melatonin
- Contributing to chronic fatigue, fibromyalgia, sleep disorders, restless leg syndrome and allergies
- Being linked with an increase in hyperactivity, depression, headaches

Researchers from the European Academy for Environmental Medicine (EUROPAEM) agree with this view, and also recommend very strict levels of Electric Fields, especially for people who are sensitive, ill, pregnant or with a compromised immunity and especially in their bedroom area at night.[396]

394 From an interview he gave to the Youtube Channel HowThingsWork. See youtube.com/watch?v=_wShp_tnjiY
395 createhealthyhomes.com
396 researchgate.net

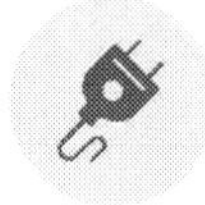

Dirty Electricity (DE)

Quick Reminder

- **Type of EMF:** Dirty Electricity (DE)
- **Measured In:** V/m (volts per meter), Graham-Stetzer (GS) units or mV (millivolts)[397]
- **Likes To:** Pollute the electricity in your house with intermediate-frequency, harmful "noise"
- **Usual Sources:** CFL and other fluorescent light bulbs, chargers for electronics, solar panel or wind turbines inverters, dimmer switches, smart appliances

Research around Dirty Electricity (DE) — remember, the intermediate, unwanted, mischievous intermediate frequencies that run on your electrical wires? — is also in its early infancy.

One thing is clear. Sam Milham, one of the world's top epidemiologists, has published serious research[398] that shows that DE can harm humans and animals alike.

Researchers from EUROPAEM report that high levels of DE in the living space have been linked in epidemiological studies to:

- Cancer
- Cardiovascular disease
- Diabetes and high blood sugar (could lead to weight gain)
- Suicide
- ADHD

Research by Magda Havas has also shown that high levels of DE can be linked with symptoms of multiple sclerosis.[399]

At the moment, there's no international standard to measure the amount of Dirty Electricity in a home or building. The Republic of Kazakhstan is the first country that has looked into the issue and taken concrete measures to reduce these levels[400] — working with electrical engineer Dave Stetzer

397 Using the Greenwave meter. See greenwavefilters.com/dirty-electricity-meter/
398 Milham, S., MD. (2012). *Dirty Electricity: Electrification and the Diseases of Civilization*. iUniverse
399 magdahavas.com
400 agriculturedefensecoalition.org

to develop special filters that do just that.

We'll get into solutions in the next pages, and I'll tell you all about these filters. In the meantime, simply understand that the less dirty the electricity in your home is, the healthier people living inside will be — especially those who are electro-sensitive.

So... What Levels of EMFs Are "Safe"?

The short answer — no one knows for sure.

The better answer — less is better.

The useful answer — keep reading.

Based on everything I've shared so far, I personally think we should try to follow the most stringent EMF safety guidelines emitted by independent experts who make it their mission to create healthier environments for their clients — like Building Biologists.[401]

This means that throughout the next Chapter, I'll show you ways you can stay within the following levels of EMF exposure:

	Radio Frequency (RF)	Magnetic Fields (MF)	Electric Fields (EF)	Dirty Electricity (DE)
Daytime	<0.2 V/m	<1 mG	<10 V/m	As low as possible
Nighttime	<0.06 V/m	<1 mG	<1.5 V/m	As low as possible
EHS People[402]	<0.02 V/m	<0.1 mG	<0.3 V/m	As low as possible

401 hbelc.org

402 Based on the advice for EHS people given out by Michael Neuert, an EMF consultant with more than 30 years of experience. These levels don't guarantee that you won't have symptoms, as people have reported being symptomatic from exposures lower than what the most sensitive EMF meters can pick up. See emfcenter.com/what-level-is-safe/

Chapter 7

WHAT TO DO

The Chapter Everyone Will Want To Skip To

How To Tame Your Phone

How To Clean Your Home

How To Protect Children

Warning: Everything I Told You So Far Is Basically Useless

After reading thousands of words about what EMFs are, how broken our current safety standards are, and how EMFs might affect your health, I'm sorry to inform you that you've gotten almost zero percent healthier — yet.

What matters now is what you'll do with the information I present in this last chapter, and how you'll change your habits around your use of technology.

So many different things emit EMFs that it gets overwhelming very quickly. To help you figure out what *your* top priorities should be, I've organized this chapter in 3 distinct sections:
Each section starts with what I call the "TTT" — Top Three Things you should do. Clever, I know.

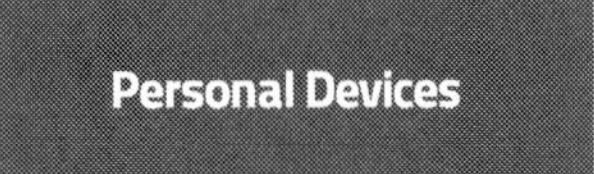

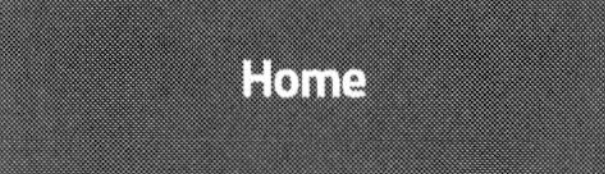

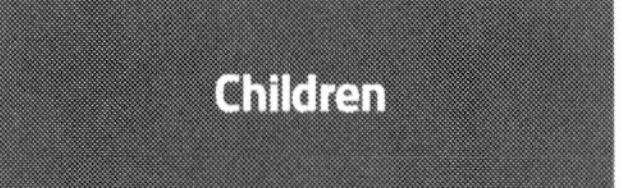

These 3 actions alone will reduce your EMF exposure by orders of magnitude, require little to no effort, and cost less than $50.

Once you implement these 3 changes into how you use technology and feel like doing more, feel free to explore the rest of the chapter. Basics first.

I've also decided to split the 3 sections above into 3 distinct levels of intervention:

Level 1: Cheap & Easy

What you can do for less than $50, and with little to no effort.

Level 2: Intermediate

Will cost more, but essential if you suffer from electro-hypersensitivity (EHS).

Level 3: EMF Expert

Never attempt on your own unless supervised by a certified Building Biologist[403] or an experienced EMF mitigation expert. You might do more harm than good.

How much should *you* do? It all depends on how sensitive you are, your budget, your resources

403 To find a Building Biologist near you, please visit hbelc.org/find-an-expert

and your motivation. But just like when it comes to any kind of environmental pollutant — the less EMFs you're exposed to, the better.

The Tool I Use To Scare Everyone Off

Activate the sound function on this thing, and you'll see people start to panic in ways you'd never expect.

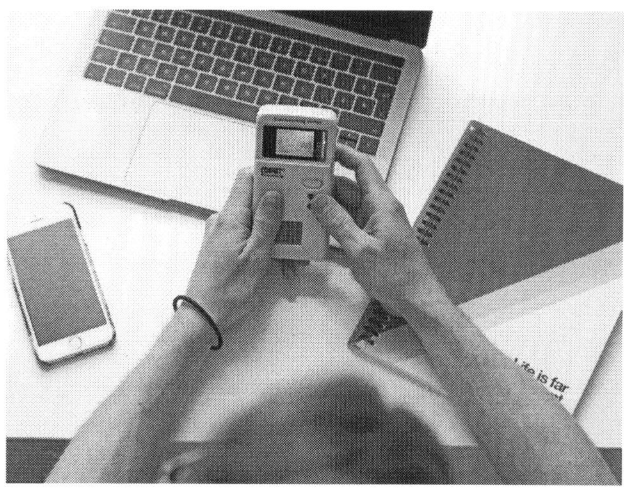

This is my Cornet ED88T Electrosmog meter — the tool I'll be using throughout this Chapter to show you how you can follow the precautionary EMF levels I've talked about on the last page of Chapter 6.

The reason I've picked this meter is that it's relatively cheap ($179 on Amazon.com), is sensitive enough to pick up concerning levels of EMFs, is easy to use and of course because it has a sound function which instantly makes everyone around you freak out.

The EMF readings I'll share with you are not scientifically accurate, because this meter isn't an engineer-level instrument. Meters of scientific precision can go up to a few thousand dollars, and unless I end up selling a trillion copies of this guide, I'll probably never buy one.

To get perfectly accurate readings in your environment, you'll have to hire a Building Biologist or EMF Expert and have them complete a home assessment that should cost you a few hundred dollars — but that I think is worth every penny.

For EMF Geeks Only
How I Measured My Numbers

I want to add this quick note for Building Biologists, doctors, EMF experts, engineers and other professionals who rightly want to make sure I understand how to use my EMF meter.

I'll be the first to admit that at the time of this writing, I'm far from having the experience of a certified Building Biologist — although I do plan to perfect my education in the field in the next years.

That being said, please note that I've taken the following into consideration when taking my measurements with the Cornet ED88T meter:

- I've decided to stick to V/m throughout this guide (instead of uW/m2), following the recommendation of Alasdair Philips, electrical engineer and founder of the advocacy group Powerwatch UK.[404]

- On most occasions, I've taken measurements at least one foot away from the source, to avoid getting overblown readings from the near-field.

- I've also made sure to move the meter around to ensure the single axis antenna was picking up signals coming off multiple directions.

- In each case, the levels I'm sharing are the highest peak values I've seen after taking a reading for at least 2 minutes. They usually don't account for obvious changes in the EMF environment on different days of the week, or different times during the day — which would have been ideal.

- To measure electric fields, I took ungrounded measurements without holding the meter in my hand. I also understand that a Cornet ED88T unfortunately doesn't go lower than 10 V/m, while the Building Biology guidelines recommend "No Anomaly" levels of 0.3 V/m at night.

- At the time of this writing, I didn't have access to a body voltage kit, which is arguably preferable (or complementary) to measure levels of electric fields in the environment.

404 powerwatch.org.uk

The Golden Rules Of EMF Mitigation

EMF experts like Daniel DeBaun and Building Biologists always stress the importance to follow these rules when trying to reduce your EMF exposure. If you don't, you'll likely do more harm than good.

Rule #1: First, Eliminate The Source

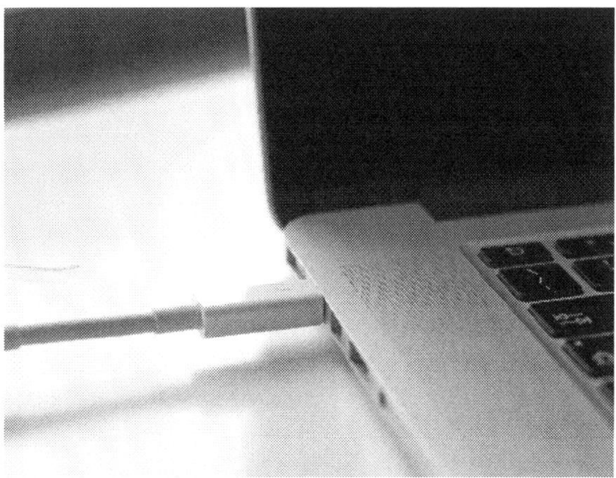

No matter how many fancy gadgets you use to "harmonize" your cell phone signals, no matter how many fancy iPhone cases you use — not using your cell phone for day-to-day communications will always be the best way to go.

The first way to reduce EMFs in your environment is to eliminate the source. For example, you could turn off the wifi function on your router at home, and use a wired connection (remember those?) instead. Problem solved.

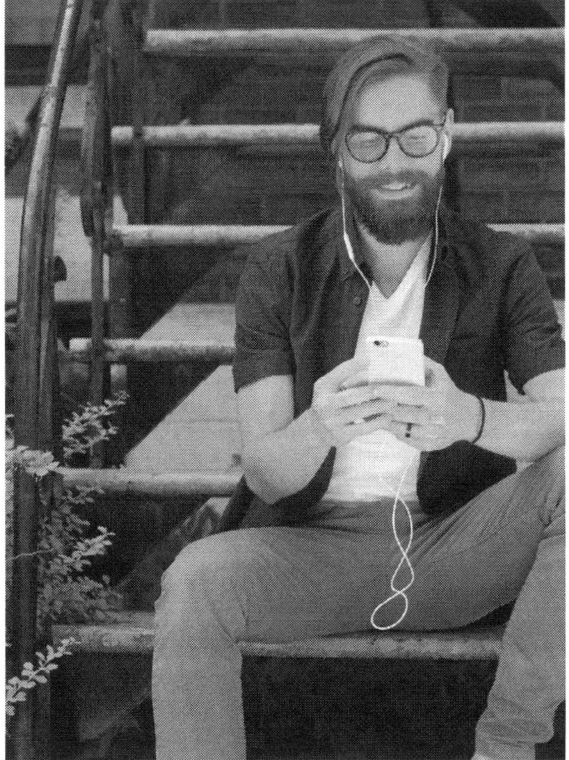

Rule #2: Increase Distance, Decrease Time

Of course, not using wifi or your cell phone is not always an option in our hyperconnected society. That's where rule #2 comes in.

If you can't eliminate the source, increase the distance between the source and your body, and decrease your time of exposure as much as possible. For example, spend less time talking on your smartphone and keep the phone at least 1 foot away from your body — using speakerphone or earbuds with an integrated microphone.

Rule #3: Shielding

If you can't eliminate the source (rule #1) and are already reducing your exposure by increasing distance and decreasing your time of use (rule #2), then we can talk about shielding — putting some kind of reflective or absorbent material between you and the source in order to reduce the levels of EMF radiation you're exposed to.

For example, it's a good idea to consider shielding your bedroom walls or windows if there happens to be a smart meter on the other side of the wall which emits constant RF radiation — but only after you've tried getting rid of the meter (the source) by asking your utility company to opt-out.

Personal Devices

Cell phones, tablets, computers, anything Bluetooth

TTT
The Three Things

1. Keep personal devices at least 1 foot from your body.

2. Make sure your computer (laptop or desktop) has a grounded 3-prong plug.

3. Reduce your use of Bluetooth devices to a minimum.

Cell Phones & Tablets - Level 1

Cheap & Easy

Some electro-sensitive people might want to get rid of their smartphone and other EMF-emitting devices altogether, but for most of us avoiding 99% of their dangers comes down to slightly changing *how* we use them.

Your cell phone or tablet is arguably the worst source of RF radiation in your life, because it's so close to your body all the time. The good news is that unlike all external sources of EMFs like smart meters, cellular antennas or even public wifi hotspots — it's also the one you have full control over.

Keep Your Devices 1 Foot Away From Your Body

It's important to understand that EMFs decrease in an exponential manner the further you get away from the source.

Distance From My iPhone 6 (4G/LTE)[405]	Peak RF Radiation (V/m)
Phone right next to head[406]	9.86
3 inches	3.7
6 inches	2.44
12 inches (1 foot)	1.42
Precautionary levels: stay under 0.2 V/m during the day.	

As you can see, distance is your friend. With every additional inch you get that device away from your body, you'll see the radiation levels drop down in a huge way.

Obviously, if you want to follow this precautionary advice and keep the device away from your body, you'll have to change your usual High-EMF habits to safer ones.

405 Measurements taken while loading a 1080p Youtube video on the 4G/LTE network, in an outside environment.

406 These readings are overblown because my EMF reader has not been engineered to measure EMFs right next to the source.

High-EMF Habits	Low-EMF Habits	Side Effect Avoided
Talking with your cell phone on your ear	Using speakerphone where appropriate, using wired earbuds while keeping the cell phone on a table instead of in your hand whenever possible	Increased cancer risks (brain, ear, salivary glands), fatigue, brain fog, eye problems, reduced neurotransmitters (depression and other neurological symptoms)
Talking for hours on your cell phone at work or at home	Redirecting your cell phone calls to a landline whenever possible	
Carrying your cell phone in your front or back pocket, in a belt holster, in your bra, or anywhere close to your body	Putting your phone on airplane mode and deactivating wifi and Bluetooth while you carry it	Increased cancer risks (close to anywhere you keep it), infertility, hormonal imbalances
	If you need to be able to take calls, putting it on a table at least 1 foot away when not in use	
Scrolling your Facebook feed while your phone is sitting on your stomach	Keeping the phone away from your intestines, especially if you have digestive issues — and sticking with games that can be played offline	Slower growth of beneficial bacteria, leaky gut, food allergies, decreased immunity, while quite possibly making candida, parasites and other opportunistic invaders much more toxic[407]

What about keeping the phone in your hand to create distance? It might be slightly better than holding it near your head or body, but my concern is that you're essentially doing is irradiating your entire blood supply (around 1.5 gallons) through the radial artery in your wrist every 60 seconds — the time it takes to complete one loop around your entire body. Not the best idea.

What about using a Bluetooth device? I'll address those in the "Anything Bluetooth" section very soon, but the short version is that they might be *slightly* better than holding a cell phone near your head, but emit the same type of EMF radiation — except even closer to your brain.

Reduce The EMF Emissions

There are also several ways to reduce how much RF radiation is emitted by your smartphone or tablet.

407 Based on the research of Dr. Dietrich Klinghardt.
See it-takes-time.com/2015/07/10/microbial-growth-and-electromagnetic-radiation/

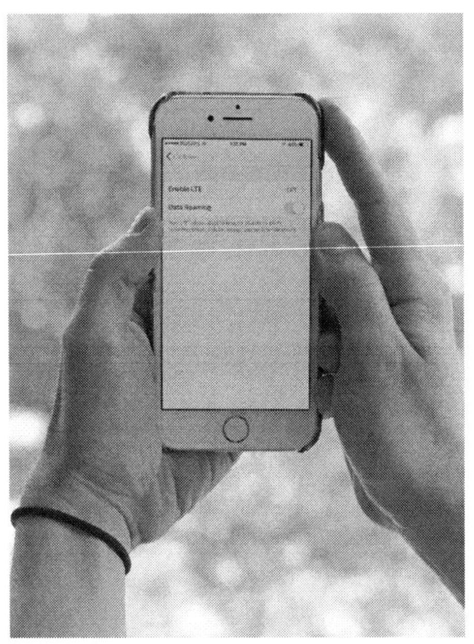

1. Disable 4G/LTE

Remember how much radiation was emitted from my iPhone 6 while downloading a YouTube video on 4G/LTE? This amount was cut down by 84% when I did the same thing using the *slightly* slower 3G network.

My trick is to keep my smartphone on 3G all the time, unless I somehow need the extra download speed (streaming video, Skype, etc.). This can be done inside your smartphone's settings.

Distance From My iPhone 6[408] (3G only)	Peak RF Radiation (V/m)
Phone right next to head[409]	1.69
3 inches	0.62
6 inches	0.38
12 inches (1 foot)	0.27
Precautionary levels: stay under 0.2 V/m during the day.	

2. Avoid Using When Reception Is Bad

As EMF activist and educator Lloyd Burrell explains, "some phones can ramp up their emissions 1000-fold in areas where the signal is poor. This means that for each signal bar that is missing your exposure increases several hundred times."[410]

Avoid using your smartphone unless you have a strong, 5/5 signal.

408 Measurements taken while loading a 1080p YouTube video on the 3G network, in an outside environment.

409 These readings are overblown because my EMF reader has not been engineered to measure EMFs right next to the source.

410 electricsense.com

3. Avoid Using In Moving Vehicles

I know, I know, there's no way you're going to stop using your cell phone to get you out of the overwhelming boredom you feel while riding the subway or bus every morning.

Still, what I'll recommend is that you put your phone on "Airplane Mode" whenever possible. Listen to podcasts, music or videos you have previously downloaded, play an offline game, and focus on stuff you can do without going online.

Unsurprisingly, the amount of EMFs you're exposing yourself to — and everyone else around — goes up tremendously when you're in a moving vehicle that's a big metal box where EMFs can happily bounce around. On top of that, radiation goes way up with poor reception, or whenever your phone needs to switch from one cell phone antenna to another throughout your ride.

Recently, I found out a way to use my iPhone 6 as a GPS while keeping it on airplane mode — which pretty much removes any reason you might have to keep your cell phone "on" while you drive.

- Disable airplane mode
- Connect to wifi or 3G to input your destination on Google Maps and pull up the itinerary
- Enable airplane mode
- Magic! Your phone can still act as a GPS!

Thanks to Apple's geolocation service that barely emits RF radiation, I'm still able to find my way around the city while avoiding 99% of the usual EMFs. I'm pretty sure this can be done with most other smartphones too.

Don't Get Fooled By Tablets

Some tablets are essentially large phones, and some phones are essentially small tablets. There's no real difference between these two devices, especially if your tablet has a SIM card which enables you to connect to the cellular network.

Everything I've said above applies to tablets too — and to desktop and laptop computers, but we'll address those two in a bit.

The biggest mistake I see when it comes to tablets is using it right in-between your legs, which is the same as telling your reproductive organs "I'm just going to microwave you a bit... okay?"

To protect your testes, spermatozoids, ovaries, eggs and especially your healthy hormone production, make sure to *never* use a tablet right next to your body either — regardless of whether you're connected to a 3G/4G network or the wifi.

Using your tablet on a large pillow will increase the distance between you and the device a bit, but will barely reduce the effects it might have on your man or lady parts. There are better solutions you can use for less than $100, if you really like surfing on the Internet your tablet while you binge on Netflix.

Cell Phones & Tablets - Level 2

Intermediate

Just in case I didn't make myself clear — everything I'll share below only applies if you're already doing every cheap & easy EMF reduction technique I've shared so far. First things first!

Use A EMF-Reducing Cell Phone Case

Don't think that a protective cell phone case will make it perfectly safe for you to talk on your cell phone for hours, right next to your head. It won't.

What it *will* do for you is to reduce the amount of EMFs your body is exposed to if you have to use a cell phone because your boss wants you to or for any other reason you personally judge important.

There are a lot of different options when it comes to phone cases, and a lot of them are either barely protective, or downright dangerous — because they block the phone's antenna and therefore force it to ramp up the radiation it emits.

The Phone Case Dilemma

I've gotten some flak from a few EMF scientists and organizations since this book was initially published, mainly over my recommendations of certain EMF-blocking products from companies such as Defender Shield, Safe Sleeve, and Belly Armor.

According to my critics, we should avoid *all* EMF-blocking products and discourage the public to buy them, on the basis that they have not been proven to work and could potentially increase people's EMF exposure (when the antenna is blocked by poor design).

While I don't agree with their point of view which I consider too reductionist, I've taken the editorial decision not to include brand recommendations inside this new edition of my book.

Instead, you can find my latest endorsements and product recommendations on my website, theeemfguy.com. I'm actively working with EMF scientists, engineers and people smarter than me to identify which products work, and which don't. My goal has always been and always will be to help you, my reader, make better choices when it comes to your health.

Finally, remember that no phone case will magically make holding a cell phone near your head 100% safe, so I still recommend using the 1-foot distance rule regardless of what cool EMF-gizmo you've proudly installed on your phone.

Use An Airtube Headset

I always use my Apple earbuds on the very rare occasions I take a phone call, but for very sensitive people or with certain types of earbuds, it might not be the best idea — because there's a possibility the metal wiring inside your headphones might act as an antenna, and transmit some of the RF signal to your brain.

I've heard conflicting reports on the subject, certain EMF experts saying that Apple earbuds are perfectly safe — and other saying they're not at all, especially for very sensitive people.

The safest option when it comes to earbuds is using what's called an "airtube headset" — which uses hollow tubes to deliver the sound to your ears instead of metal wiring, removing any possibility of EMFs running up the wire.

They also reduce the otherwise-inevitable exposure you'd get to the low level Magnetic Fields emitted by any kind of speaker — which gets worse the more you crank up the volume.

Another option recommended by Building Biologist Oram Miller is to install a $5 small ferrite bead on your headphone's wire. Problem solved.

Use An EMF-Harmonizing Chip

I warn you — this part is going to get pretty woo-woo.

The second you start Googling around to find ways to reduce the dangers of EMFs, you come across dozens and dozens of different EMF-harmonizing devices, created by dozens of companies each claiming their device is the ultimate solution to make your cell phone safe again.

The way these devices are said to work is by harmonizing (not reducing) the EMFs coming off your device, which could potentially make this radiation more compatible with the human body.

There are a ton of different technologies which might all have their merits, but for simplicity's sake everything I'll tell you here applies to any EMF-harmonizing device that is said to work through:

Sacred Geometry	Harmonizing Energies	Crystals
Scalar Energy	Subtle Energy	Orgonite
Shungite	Pulsed Electromagnetic Fields (PEMF)	Coherent Field Generators
Schumann Frequency Generators	Biogeometry	Chi Energy

I fully intend to dive deeper in the subject in the future, because there are thousands of testimonials and dozens of well-designed studies showing the efficacy of some of these products in reducing symptoms of electro-hypersensitivity (EHS), even when placebo-controlled.

That being said, all this research is still so unclear that I've decided to stick once again with the recommendations made by Building Biologists,[411] which are:

1. Do not use subtle energy devices as a sole means of protection, or even as your first line of protection against EMFs.

2. Use them as supplemental protection against electromagnetic radiation in situations where it cannot be avoided.

3. Use them as an adjunct to EMF reduction/elimination strategies in your living and work spaces, particularly for people with electrical sensitivity.

4. Put into practice methods that will eliminate or reduce exposure to EMF radiation in spaces that you control.

I agree with the position of Oram Miller and researcher Magda Havas, who both recommend people to only invest in stickers, pendants, chips and other EMF-harmonizing devices that offer a money-back guarantee.

If the devices do nothing to make your sleep better or to lessen your electrosensitivity, simply ask for your money back.

---

411 In their 2015 position paper. See hbelc.org/pdf/standards/SEDs_v1.12.pdf

Recommended Products

Our global understanding of EMF science and engineering evolves very quickly, and it is a real challenge to assess which gizmos are really worth your time and money. To get my latest endorsements and product recommendations, please visit theeemfguy.com

Computers - Level 1

Cheap & Easy

Next to your smartphone or tablets, computers (laptop or desktop) are definitely a huge source of RF radiation when connected via wifi and/or Bluetooth, and a huge source of Magnetic Fields which are emitted by the hard drive and power supply.

Just like your smartphone or tablet, these are cool EMF-emitting gadgets that we all need to use in a smarter way.

Emits RF & MF Levels From My MacBook Pro

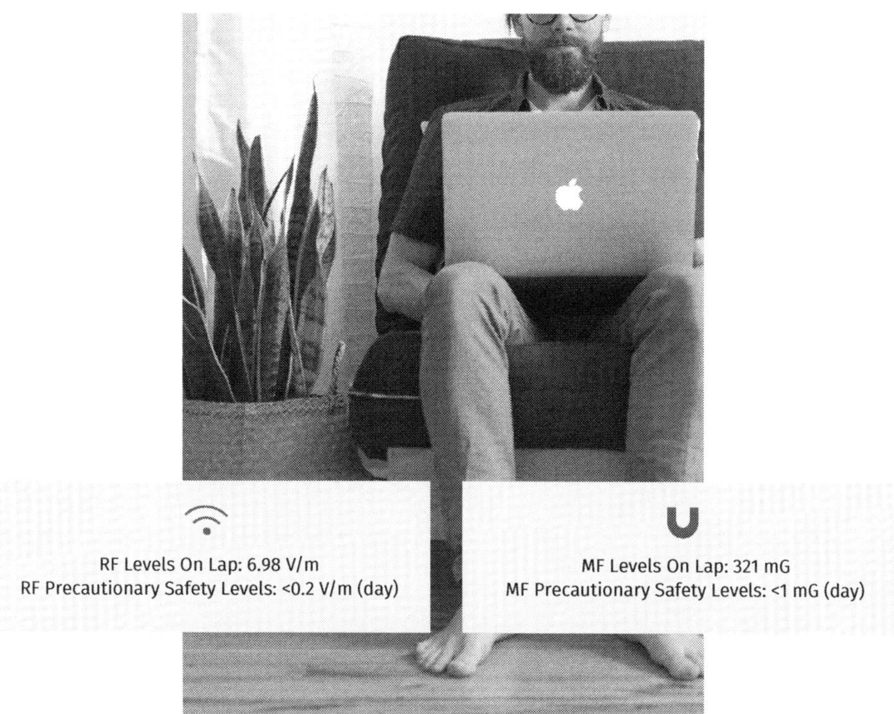

RF Levels On Lap: 6.98 V/m
RF Precautionary Safety Levels: <0.2 V/m (day)
MF Levels On Lap: 321 mG
MF Precautionary Safety Levels: <1 mG (day)

Keep Your Computer At Least 1 Foot Away From Your Body

Believe it or not, laptops were never meant to be used on your lap. As reported in *Radiation Nation*,[412] "the first laptop computer, designed in 1979, actually weighed twenty-four pounds and was created to be placed on a desk." Thanks to our incredible advances in technology, however,

412 DeBaun, D. and DeBaun, R. (2017). *Radiation Nation: The Fallout of Modern Technology — Your Complete Guide to EMF Protection & Safety: The Proven Health Risks of Electromagnetic Radiation (EMF) & What to Do Protect Yourself & Family*. Icaro Publishing.

we now have laptops that weigh less than two pounds — and that sit perfectly on your thighs.

The problem is that your laptop emits a ton of RF radiation (similar frequencies as cell phones) when connected to wifi.

A better option to save your fertility would be to use your laptop on a table — your IKEA pillow won't cut it!

If you're particularly sensitive to EMFs, you might want to create even more distance between you and your laptop. I personally use a Roost Stand (combined with an external keyboard and mouse) in an honest attempt to both save my posture and create more distance between me and my laptop.

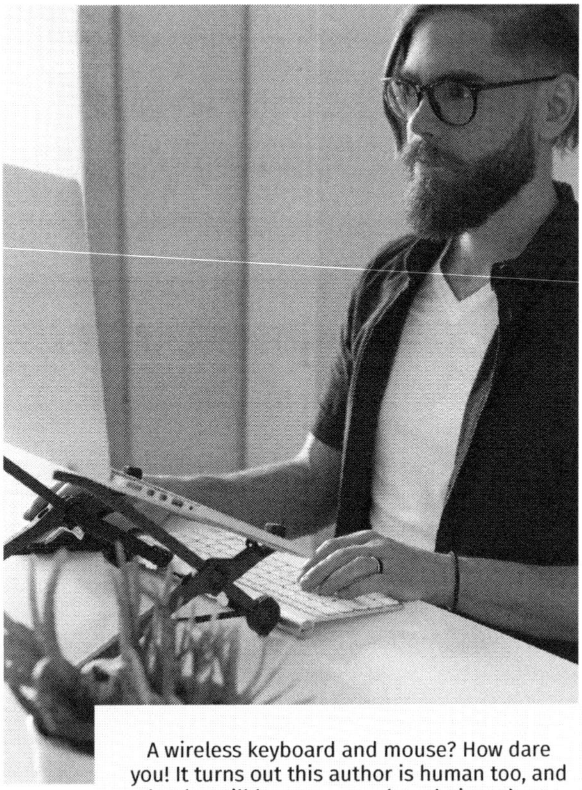

A wireless keyboard and mouse? How dare you! It turns out this author is human too, and that he still has some work to do in order to minimize his EMF exposure.

Go Wired

In case you forgot, just a few years ago there was no such thing as wifi. In these old, dark times, people actually had to plug their computer to a router in order to go online. I swear.

If you want to keep your EMF exposure to a minimum, wired is still the way to go. It's faster, more secure, more stable, and safer for your body.

You can use a wired connection on virtually any device, even though it's becoming more complicated since most electronics manufacturers have started removing standard Ethernet sockets from most computers.

How To Go Wired	
Laptop computer	Use a standard RJ45 connector, or use the appropriate converter if your computer has no Ethernet socket
Tablet Smartphone	Google around for a tutorial on how to use wired Internet on your specific device. Here's one for the iPad[413]

If you choose to go completely wired, remember to visit the settings of your router and to shut down the wifi function. Even if there are no devices connected to the router, it will still be emitting RF radiation 24/7 unless you do so.

Make Sure Your Computer Is Grounded

If you have a desktop computer, this shouldn't be a problem. But if you have a laptop, this can be a huge issue that's going to sap your energy and mental power.

Most computer chargers are grounded by default. If yours has a 3-prong connection, it means that it's grounded.

However, if the cord only has 2 prongs, it means that your laptop will be a huge source of Electric Fields (EF) — and that you'll essentially get zapped with low-level electrical shocks all day (without feeling them) while you type away at the keyboard.

Grounded

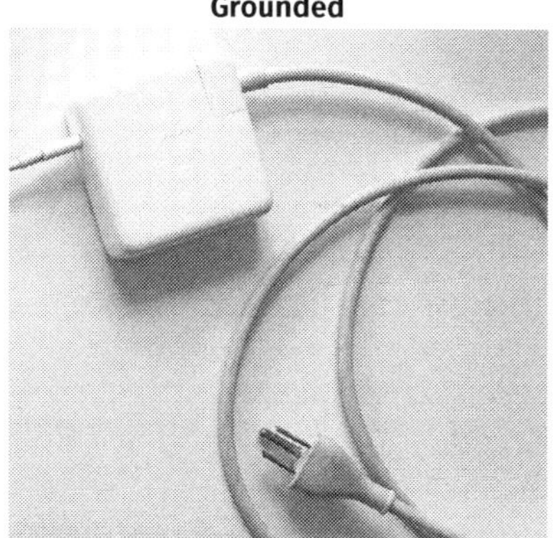

Ungrounded

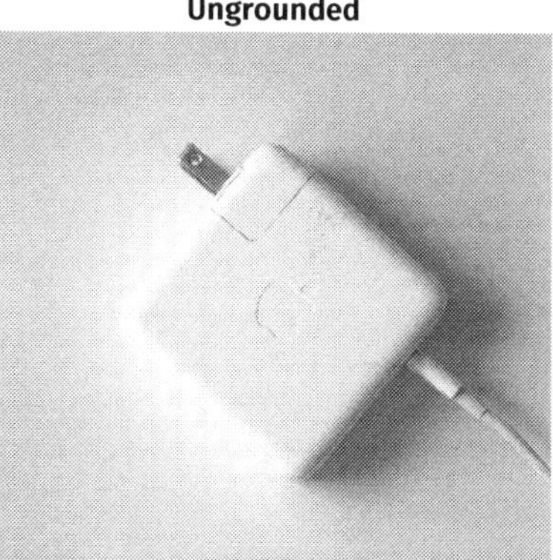

In one case study,[414] EMF mitigation specialist Michael Neuert found that just the act of standing in front of an ungrounded computer was transferring 1.9 volts of stray electric energy through his body (body voltage method), which is 190 times higher than levels considered perfectly safe by Building Biologists.

This will be a recurring theme throughout this Chapter. Grounded electronics = good. Ungrounded electronics = bad idea, and a huge source of energy-sapping Electric Fields (EF).

413 lifewire.com
414 See youtube.com/watch?v=33kTot8IBws

How To Make Sure Your Computer Is Grounded

1. Make sure the charger has 3 prongs.

2. If it has two prongs, you can use a special USB ground cord which connects your computer to the ground in a wall outlet[415]

3. Bonus points if you use an outlet tester to make sure the outlet's ground works properly[416]

4. If you can't ground your laptop right now, use it on battery power, and recharge it when not in use

Organize Your Cords & Chargers

There's a very strong reason you'll want to organize your cords and chargers, and it's not just because you want your workspace to be Instagram-ready.

Let me go back to what I explained at the very beginning of this guide about the difference between Electric Fields (EF) and Magnetic Fields (MF) — using the analogy of a garden hose.

- **When water (electricity) is flowing out of the hose, it creates MF radiation around the source — in that case, around your charger.**

- **The pressure of water (electricity) inside the hose creates large electric fields around the hose (wires), which can transfer to your body.**

In plain English, it means two things: don't keep your feet or legs right next to your chargers or any wiring, or you'll be exposed to huge sources of unnecessary EMFs — which can drain your energy, trigger other symptoms in sensitive people, or simply leave you with a nice headache right in the middle of your work day.

---

415 See lessemf.com/ground.html (costs $9)
416 See amazon.com (costs $9)

EMF Levels From My MacBook Pro Charger[417]

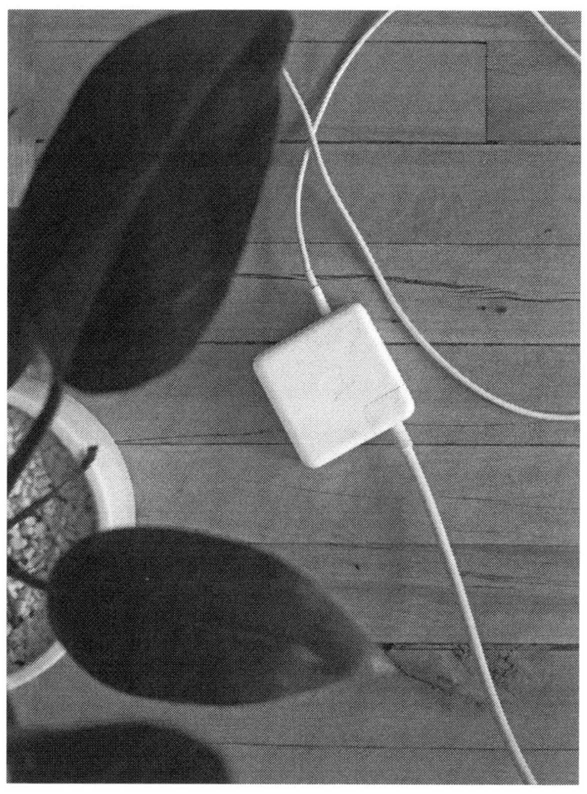

Electric Fields
(always inside the cord even when not in use)

EF Levels Right Next To Charger: 444 V/m
EF Precautionary Safety Levels: <10 V/m (day)

Magnetic Fields
(only present while it's charging)

MF Levels Right Next To Charger: 467 mG
MF Precautionary Safety Levels: <1 mG (day)

This bears the question... what distance should you keep between you and your computer cords or charger?

One foot is the very minimum and should make you avoid most of the Magnetic Fields, but Electric Fields are usually way larger than that — so tucking your wires at least 3 feet away from where your feet are is a good idea.

417 Both of these numbers will be overblown because of the lack of sensitivity of my meter very close to the source. For reference only.

Computers - Level 2

Intermediate

If you already use a wired connection whenever possible, never put a laptop on your lap, and make sure your computer is grounded — I don't have much else to tell you.

Remember that if you insist on using a computer on your lap, placing a large pillow or cushion between you and the computer will still blast your sexual organs with large amounts of RF radiation at levels shown to affect your fertility.

If you insist on using your laptop connected on wifi (hey, some people still make the conscious decision to keep smoking after all) — then at least look into an EMF-shielding solution[418] like a Belly Armor Blanket.[419]

It would be a huge mistake to think that a blanket will completely protect you, because we don't have the science to prove that. In the end, consider EMF-shielding products like smoking "lighter" cigarettes. Might be a bit better for you but in the end it's still smoking.

Recommended Products

Our global understanding of EMF science and engineering evolves very quickly, and it is a real challenge to assess which gizmos are really worth your time and money. To get my latest endorsements and product recommendations, please visit theeemfguy.com

418 You can find my latest product endorsements and recommendations at theemfguy.com

419 No need to be pregnant to use this one. I've heard reports of Silicon Valley executives using it all day while working at their laptop.

Anything Bluetooth

My advice when it comes to using any Bluetooth device near your body is this — less is better.

Generally, Bluetooth devices emit very low levels of RF radiation, which is a good thing. However, they are also worn very close to the body, and 24/7 in the case of certain wearables — so they can be a huge issue.

Avoid "Class 1" Devices.

As EMF activist Lloyd Burrell explains,[420] Bluetooth devices are organized in 3 classes:

Bluetooth Class	Range (in ft)	Power (in mW)
1	300	100
2	33	2.5
3	<33	1

Class 3 devices emit 100 times less EMFs than class 1 devices, which makes them an obvious choice. Unfortunately, manufacturers are currently not required to disclose which class of Bluetooth their device uses, and how much radiation they emit. Make sure to do your research and contact the manufacturer before purchasing anything.

For your cell phone, I still recommend using earbuds over a Bluetooth earpiece, but if you insist on using Bluetooth — here's a list of known "Class 2" ear pieces:[421]

- Plantronics Voyager Legend
- Plantronics Backbeat
- Motorola S305 Bluetooth Stereo Headset
- LanAuBluetooth Headphones
- Avantree Bluetooth Over Ear Headphones

If you ignore this advice and just buy a random earpiece, be warned that it could technically expose your brain to much more radiation than your cell phone itself.[422]

420 electricsense.com
421 As Burrell points out, older Class 3 ear pieces have unfortunately been phased out and replaced with more powerful Class 2 devices.
422 In one case, EMF expert Michael Neuert reports having measured levels of RF radiation emitted by a Bluetooth earpiece which were 7 times higher than the levels emitted by a cell phone. Yikes.

Use Wearables You Can Put On "Airplane Mode".

Manufacturers of health-tracking devices are starting to wake up to consumer demand, and some offer the option to turn off the Bluetooth function inside their product on demand — which means you simply have to turn it back on whenever you need to sync your data.

If you find a device that you love but that emits radiation 24/7 — get in touch with the company, and let them know you want the option to turn the Bluetooth off! The more demand there is, the faster manufacturers will listen and start offering better and safer products.

Anything Metallic

I really didn't know where to put this part — but it's also very important to talk about how wearing anything metallic in and out of your body might act as an antenna and attract some of the EMFs in your environment.

	Concern	Solution
Tattoos	Heavy metals used in the ink are known to react to MRIs[423] and some think they might react to EMFs in the environment too	Opt for metal-free inks. Do your research!
Metal-frame glasses	Wearing metal-frame glasses might make cell phone radiation stronger[424]	Opt for plastic or wood-frame glasses
Dental amalgams or fixtures	Amalgams leach more mercury when exposed to cell phones[425] and wifi[426]	Find a biological dentist who knows how to safely remove dental amalgams[427]
Shielded clothing	Can do more harm than good and actually make your EMF exposure worse[428]	Stick with reputable companies and always test your before/after using an EMF meter
Bras with a metal underwire	The link between bras underwires and breast cancer is still unclear, but not impossible[429]	Bras with no underwire[430]
Metal jewelry	Some people who suffer from severe electrohypersensitivity (EHS) report getting sicker when wearing metal on their body[431]	Stick with non-metallic jewelry if this is your case

423 livescience.com
424 ncbi.nlm.nih.gov/pubmed/18003202
425 ncbi.nlm.nih.gov/pubmed/18819554
426 ncbi.nlm.nih.gov/pmc/articles/PMC4944481
427 To find a Biological Dentist, visit iaomt.org/search/
428 See Lloyd Burrell's article on the subject: electricsense.com/9354/emf-shielded-clothing-work/
429 The strongest hypothesis is that bras might reduce the lymphatic circulation in your breasts, but it's not implausible that a metal underwire could also increase the amount of EMFs absorbed by your breast tissue. See breastcancerconqueror.com/take-off-your-bra/ and emfacts.com/2005/11/breast-cancer-and-microwaves/
430 Ironically, these are often called "wireless" bras.
431 weepinitiative.org

Home

Creating Your Low-EMF Haven

TTT
The Three Things

1. Turn Off Anything-Wifi At Night

2. Shut Down The Circuit Breakers For Your Bedroom (Or Entire House) At Night

3. Get Rid Of CFL Light Bulbs, Baby Monitors And Cordless Phones

Creating Your Low-EMF Haven

How do you feel when you leave the city for a few days and spend time in nature? Pretty good? Calmer? Centered? Alive?

I'm (and hundreds of experts I told you about throughout this guide) convinced that one of the reasons we feel that way is because these environments are usually very low in background EMFs.[432]

Reducing the EMFs in your home environment where you spend at least a third of your day will certainly do no harm, and chances are it'll improve your health in every way possible.

In the last few years, investor and EMF activist Peter Sullivan has set up a special low-EMF tent at the Autism One conference where he speaks on the link between EMFs and autism.

He reports that a vast majority of people who visit the tent feel an instant difference in how they feel.[433] They report being calmer, more centered. But for sensitive people, the experience can even be life-changing.

One woman's Tourette syndrome went away within 20 minutes of entering the tent. The same thing happened with someone who had been suffering from tinnitus (ringing in the ears) for years. Autistic children become less agitated, and literally fall asleep right there, on the ground — and you can almost hear their body say "dude... I've been waiting for this loud noise to stop my entire life!"

Warning: Overwhelm Right Ahead

I remember the overwhelm I personally felt when I started to uncover the different sources of EMFs in my living space — the tiny apartment I share with my wife and business partner Geneviève in Montreal.

Smart meters. 20 different wifi networks I could detect with my iPhone. Old, quite possibly faulty wiring. Cell towers? Where are these things again? What if I can't see them, but they're still blasting away at my skull while I sleep? What about my own wifi router... is it far enough from my pillow?

432 Unfortunately, there are so many cellular towers being installed in the countryside that low-EMF environments should probably be classified as protected species.

433 youtube.com

Luckily for you, I spent enough time researching EMF solutions (not just problems) that this next part should empower you instead of leaving you paranoiac and fearful.

I'll let you know what your top priorities should be inside your home environment, whatever your situation happens to be, and then go room-by-room to teach you what can be done to reduce EMFs.

Again, I'll put the cheap & easy solutions first, followed by more expensive and demanding (but better) interventions. I'll also tell you in which situations I recommend hiring a Building Biologist or EMF mitigation expert to test the levels in your environment and provide advanced, engineer-level solutions to your EMF problem.

The 6 Most Worrisome EMF Sources At Home

Wifi Router	**Sneaky Sources Of Wifi**	**Circuit Breaker Panel**
Dirty Electricity	**Wiring Errors**	**Current On Water Or Gas Pipes**

Wifi Router - Level 1

Cheap & Easy

Remember the first golden rule of EMF mitigation? Eliminate the source. If you suffer from electro-hypersensitivity or want to create a very low-EMF home, you'll have to get rid of your wifi router and go the old-fashioned way — 100% wired.

If that's not possible, we need to look at rule #2 — increase distance, and decrease time. Every solution I'll share below will help you do just that.

Move That Router Away

Your #1 mission is to get your wifi router as far away from your living spaces as possible — all while being able to get a signal just good enough to prevent you from losing your darn mind over connectivity problems, which in some people I think could literally be worse than the EMFs themselves.

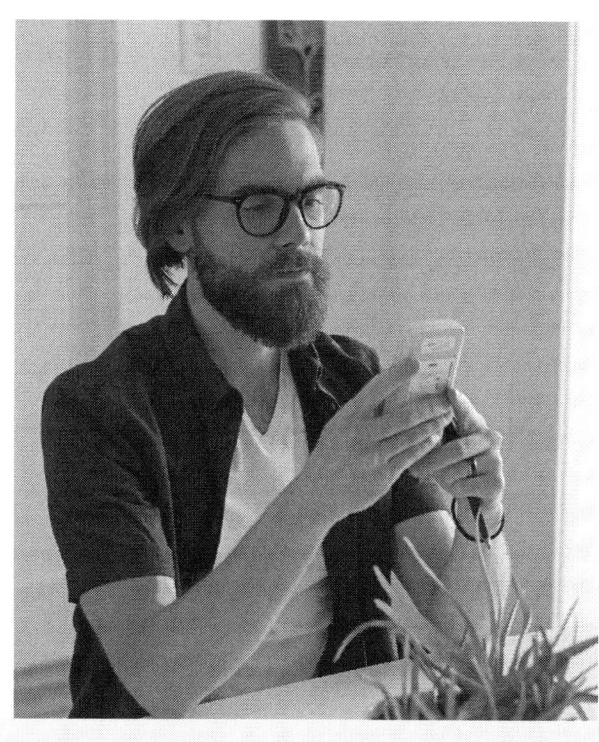

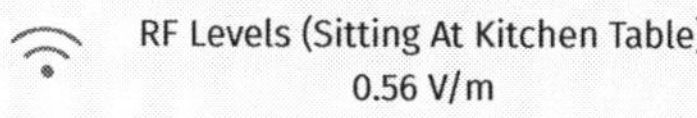

RF Levels (Sitting At Kitchen Table)
0.56 V/m

RF Precautionary Safety Levels
<0.2 V/m (day)

Unfortunately, I live in a relatively small space, which means my router is sitting 4-5 feet from the kitchen table.

If you live in a large city and can detect 120 different wifi networks around you (all with different, sometimes vulgar and often surprisingly creative names), don't worry too much — there's little you can do about your neighbors, and your own wifi router is emitting levels thousands of times higher because of its proximity.

The further away you get from that thing, the better. I know you want a precise number — so let's go with the recommendation given by the authors of *Radiation Nation*,[434] which is to keep

434 DeBaun, D. and DeBaun, R. (2017). *Radiation Nation: The Fallout of Modern Technology — Your Complete Guide to EMF Protection & Safety: The Proven Health Risks of Electromagnetic Radiation (EMF) & What to Do Protect Yourself & Family*. Icaro Publishing.

at least 10 feet between your body and your router.

Keep in mind that wifi goes through walls pretty easily, so don't think the 10-feet rule doesn't apply to you if the router is in a different room.

Shut It Down When Not In Use

Most people are so used to having their wifi router "ON" 24/7 that they even start to wonder if it's safe to turn it off when not in use, or if it's going to break the Internetz.

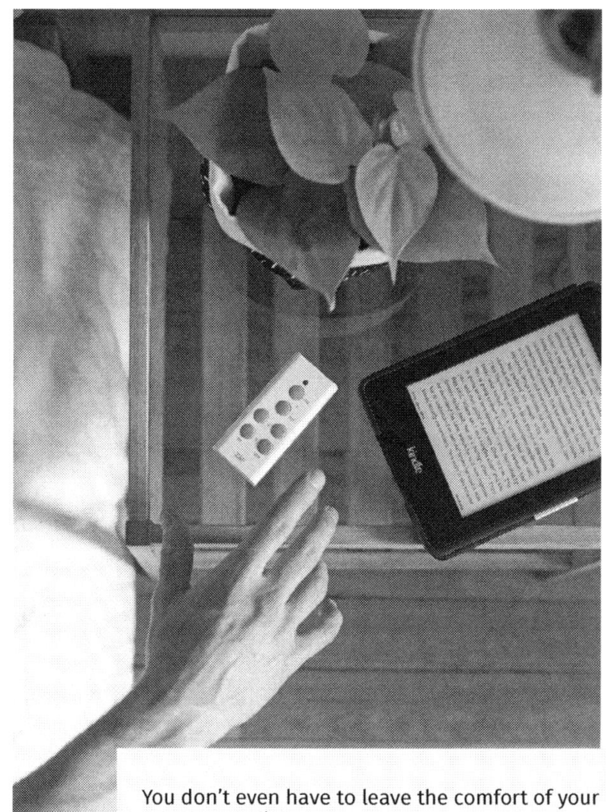

You don't even have to leave the comfort of your bed. Just click, turn off that nasty router, and sleep like a baby.

Don't worry, unplugging your router won't do anything bad. Instead, it might just reduce your electricity bill a bit, and definitely give your body a well-deserved break from all these signals.

The most important time to unplug your wifi router is at night — where you really shouldn't be still awake scrolling your Facebook or Instagram feed anyway, and where a high-EMF environment will cause the most harm by preventing your body from getting into a deep, restorative, REM sleep stage.

If you're not the last person in your household going to bed, install the same kind of plug-in timer you'd use for Christmas lights or remote-controlled outlets like the ones I got off Amazon.

I'll share all my brands recommendations in the "Recommended Products" section below.

Reduce The Power

Under the admin settings of certain wifi routers,[435] you can reduce the power of the signal, or

435 If you have no idea of what I'm talking about, read this tutorial on how to access your router's

"signal strength". You can try playing around with the setting, and lower it down to a level good enough for you to get online. You'll dramatically reduce the amount of EMFs it's emitting.

In these settings, you'll also find the option to turn the wifi signal off altogether. If you decide to use a wired connection throughout your home, use this option. Unlike what most people think, the wireless signal won't stop being emitted when you connect a wire to your router.

Turn Off The Public Wifi

What public wifi? The somewhat hidden public wifi that certain Internet providers have started installing in the wifi routers they've been giving their clients in the last few years.

Since 2013 in the US of A, Comcast has been executing its "monster project to blanket the entire nation with continuous wifi coverage."[436] And in order to do this, Comcast distributes wifi routers that automatically create a public wifi network inside your home, emitting EMFs 24/7 for the online enjoyment of your neighbors and random people walking down the street while playing Angry Birds.

I've heard multiple reports of people having a real hard time turning off this public wifi. In multiple cases, the wifi was still emitting inside their house even after Comcast assured them multiple times that this option had been turned off on their end.

If you have a wifi router from any of the companies below,[437] make sure to call them and turn the public wifi off. If you have a EMF meter, that's even better — you'll be able to confirm that they did turn it off.

North America: Comcast, Cablevision

Europe: BT, UPC, Virgin, XLN

Unfortunately, the phenomenon of sneaking public wifi into private routers is becoming widespread. One study by Juniper Research found that a third of all routers sold in the US had public wifi at the beginning of 2017.[438]

---

settings using any web browser: pcmag.com/article/346184/how-to-access-your-wifi-routers-setting

436 money.cnn.com

437 These lists are probably incomplete, and new companies are joining the trend every year.

438 slate.com

Wifi Router - Level 2

Intermediate

The JRS Eco-Wifi Firmware (Installed On An Asus Router)

While virtually every single electrical engineer in the world seems to be focused on designing wifi routers with faster speed, more coverage and more aggressive connectivity — one man has developed what's probably the first and only "low-EMF"[439] router.

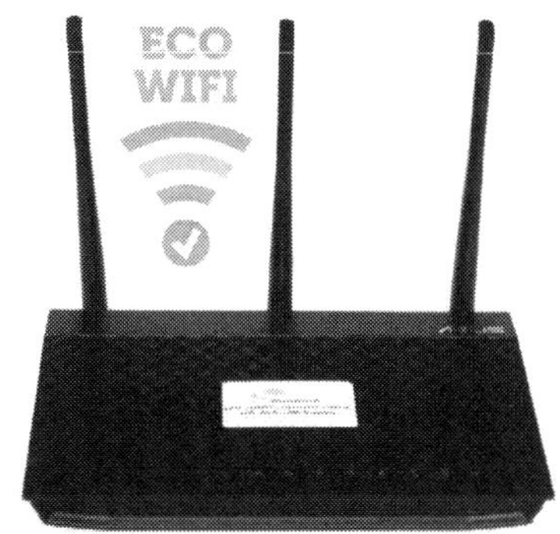

Dr. Jan-Rutger Schrader, PhD, has successfully engineered a wifi router which offers a technically measurable reduction in EMF emissions, without reducing its speed or coverage.

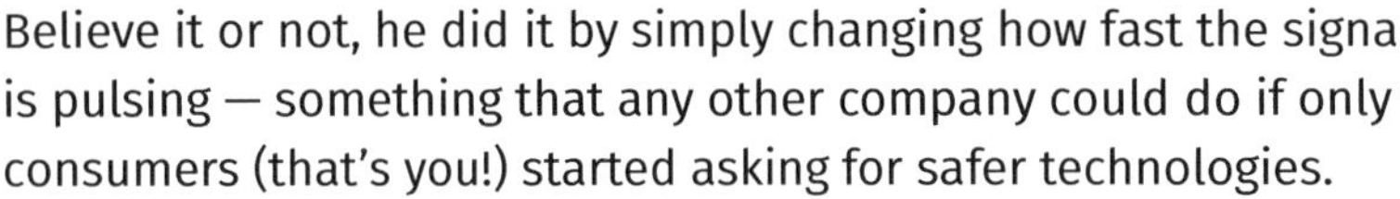

Believe it or not, he did it by simply changing how fast the signal is pulsing — something that any other company could do if only consumers (that's you!) started asking for safer technologies.

Dr. Schrader says you can use this wifi router with virtually any Internet service provider around the world, but I'd make sure to contact his customer service team before making the investment, just to be sure.

Using A Router Guard

If you can't manually decrease the power output of your wifi router, another option is to put your router inside a shielded "Router Guard", which acts as a small Faraday cage.[440] This will both cut down on the EMF emissions, but also on the speed of your connection. Might be a good option if you live in a small house or apartment.

439 Even if this router emits lower amounts of EMFs, I wouldn't recommend standing right next to it or keeping it turned on at night.

440 A Faraday cage or Faraday shield is an enclosure used to block electromagnetic fields.

Recommended Products

Our global understanding of EMF science and engineering evolves very quickly, and it is a real challenge to assess which gizmos are really worth your time and money. To get my latest endorsements and product recommendations, please visit theeemfguy.com

Sneaky Sources Of Wifi - Level 1

Cheap & Easy

Aside from the very sneaky public wifi that's installed on a third of all private routers, there are a ton of electronics in your home that constantly emit invisible RF signals right under your nose. How rude.

As companies continue to push the idea of a smart, hyperconnected home and the Internet of Things (IoT) — where everything ranging from your light switches to your plants will be connected to the Internet — it will become harder and harder to identify these sources of EMFs unless you have a meter like mine, or hire an EMF expert to do a home assessment (always highly recommended).

Scrap The Baby Monitor

How can I put this bluntly? If you put a baby monitor in your child's crib, you might as well use a 4G phone instead — because certain monitors are essentially small cellular antennas.

In a 2014 interview given to CBS 2 Local News,[441] Building Biologist Oram Miller measured levels of 6.14 V/m (in RF radiation) being emitted at close range from a baby monitor — that's 102X more than the precautionary levels we're trying to achieve of 0.06 V/m at night.

Jump to the "Children" section to learn about safer options for baby monitors.

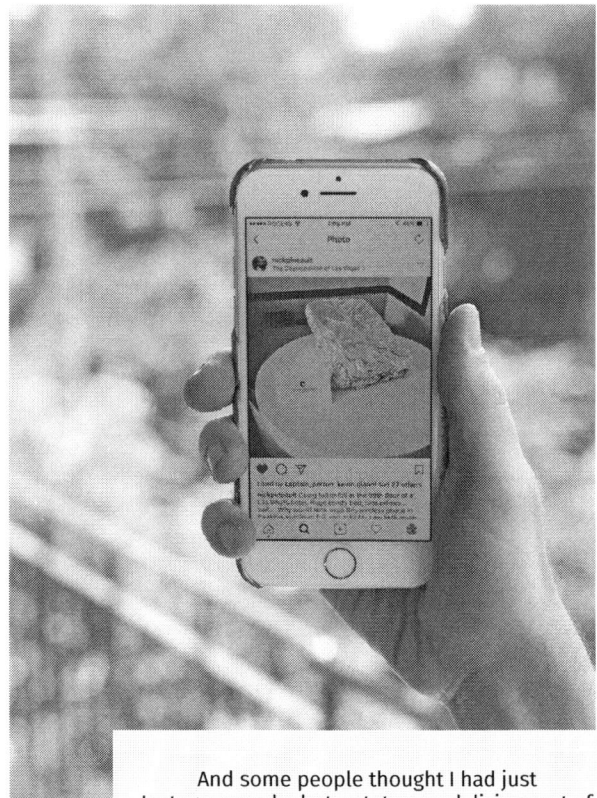

And some people thought I had just Instagrammed a hot potato or a delicious set of PB&J sandwiches. I understand the confusion.

Scrap Your Cordless Phones

One type of cordless phone — called the "DECT" (Digital Enhanced Cordless Telecommunications) phone — is way worse than any cell phone, wifi router or baby

441 youtube.com

monitor, combined.

The power will vary from model to model, but unless you possess (or rent) an EMF meter or hire an EMF expert to verify exactly how much of an issue yours is... I'd highly advise getting rid of the wireless phones in your home.

In a beautiful room at the Aria hotel in Vegas, unaware interior designers thought that putting a DECT phone right next to my comfy bed would be the perfect addition to a luxury experience.

But when my EMF meter read peaks of 26 V/m right next to it... I knew I would wake up hungover even without having even one overpriced cocktail. I ended up going "full tinfoil" and literally wrapped the whole thing in aluminum foil,[442] which reduced the levels to around 0.32 V/m at 2 feet. Way better.

Unplug Everything "Smart" Or That Uses Wifi (When Not In Use)

If you're trying to create a healthy low-EMF environment at home, your smart devices are actually pretty stupid — in the sense that most of them send pulses of RF signals all day, every day — even when turned off.

Let me repeat it again so it sinks in... they keep emitting signals even when you click the big OFF button.

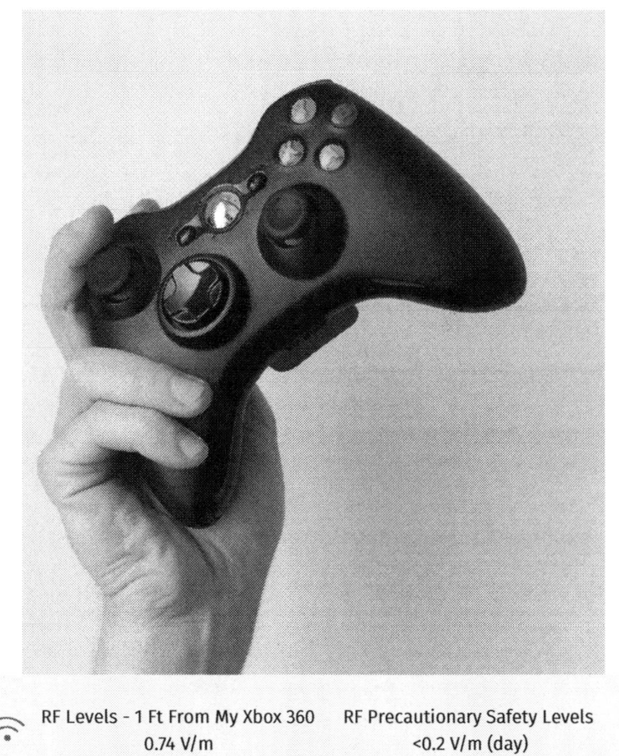

RF Levels - 1 Ft From My Xbox 360: 0.74 V/m — RF Precautionary Safety Levels: <0.2 V/m (day)

I was stunned when I realized that our Xbox 360 is trying to connect to the wifi router 24/7, unless I completely unplug it. This means during the 23 hours per day I'm not using the device, I'm still being exposed to a source of 100% useless radiation.

Brand new "smart" appliances also

442 Aluminum foil is actually a great shielding material for RF radiation, which is the idea behind electro-sensitive people wearing a "tinfoil hat".

connect to new wireless "smart" utility meters, sometimes several times every second, all day, every day — in order to communicate information about how much electricity it's using, when you're opening the fridge, when you're doing the laundry, etc.[443]

The same is true for most (read: probably all) smart TVs, which nowadays don't even offer the option to shut down their connectivity to wifi or Bluetooth inside their settings.

On top of that — in a bold 1984-esque move, Samsung also recommends its own customers not to discuss personal information in front of their smart TV (yes, even when turned off), because the information you share *will* be sold to a 3rd party if you have the the voice-activated feature turned on.[444]

The lesson here? Make sure that these things are also unplugged at night, and minimize the amount of smart devices you have at home as much as possible.

Common "Smart" Devices That Emit 24/7 RF Signals

Smart TVs & Other Appliances	Apple TV, Roku & Other Media Players	Bluetooth Dimmer Switches
Bluetooth Speakers & Thermostats	Video Game Consoles	Wireless Anything!

443 See this video demonstration from EMF activist Lloyd Burrell: youtube.com/watch?v=yqomG3xmAcQ
444 It does sound like conspiracy-theory-level BS, but it's really not. theweek.com

Sneaky Sources Of Wifi - Level 3

EMF Expert

I won't repeat this part every single time, but understand that any issue I'm talking about in this chapter can be better taken care of when you work with a certified Building Biologist or EMF expert.

These guys have a ton of experience, operate professional-level meters, and can help you detect and reduce EMFs in your home environment better than I could ever show you inside this introductory-level guide.

Main Breaker Panel

This one is going to be short and sweet.

If your main breaker panel is far, far away (more than 10 feet) from your living spaces, skip this part. But if it's very close to your bedroom or somewhere your children play, we've got a problem.

Anytime you're in a presence of a strong electrical transformer, you can bet there are strong levels of Magnetic Fields (MF) around.

Luckily, the levels drop very rapidly with distance, so like I said your main circuit breaker panel shouldn't be much of an issue unless it's right next to a living space or right on the other side of your bedroom's wall — in which case you'll have to hire a EMF expert to measure the levels and make sure your environment is actually safe.

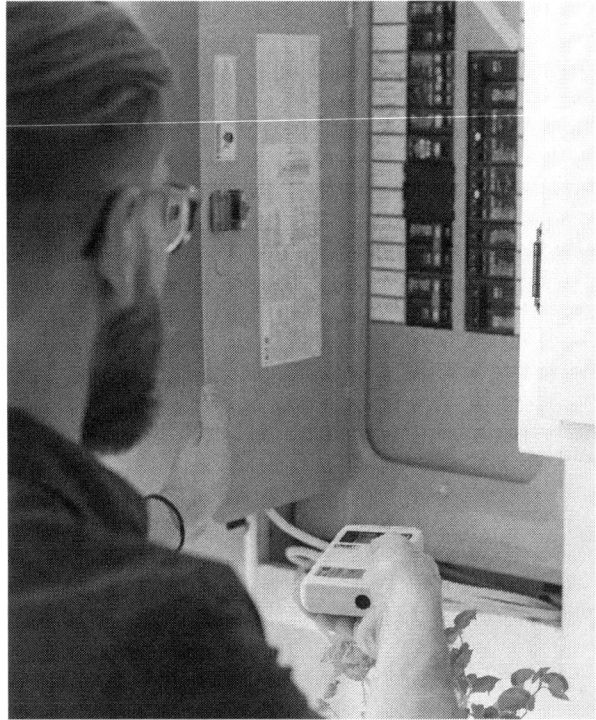

	MF Levels - 1 Ft From Breaker Panel 3.3 mG	MF Precautionary Safety Levels <1 mG (day)

Dirty Electricity (DE)

Quick reminder — dirty electricity is essentially the measure of how clean the electricity running inside your home is.

The dirtier the electricity in your home is, the more harmful Electric Fields (EF)[445] will be radiating from the standard wiring in the walls. And for most people, this exposure to very high levels of DE will rhyme with unstable blood sugar, less deep sleep, ADHD, depression and fatigue.

This is where I'll get a lot of flak from some people in the EMF community. But what the heck... I'm here to tell you what I consider to be the truth, inconvenient or not.

When you Google around for ways to reduce the dirty electricity in a home, you instantly come across what are called "dirty electricity filters" — plug-in devices that are said to take care of the problem. Just plug around 20 of these devices (which would cost you around $700) around your home, and you're all set.

As reported by Dr. Magda Havas and electrical engineer Dave Stetzer,[446] doing just that — using special filters to reduce levels of DE — has lead to incredible recoveries in people suffering from EHS, healing responses in diabetics, a reduction in symptoms of ADHD in kids, and much more. So far, so good.

But there's also a darker side to the story. In some cases, very sensitive people seem to get *worse* when the filters are installed. In some other cases — like when installed in a house that has wiring errors — these filters can create incredibly high levels of Magnetic Fields (MF) in the living area.

Enter Michael Schwaebe

I just couldn't settle for a solution that can potentially help some people, but hurt others. It simply doesn't make sense.

After much research, I decided to contact Michael Schwaebe, a veteran Building Biologist who published a lot of information on the subject. Michael generously offered to get on the (corded) phone and help me to write this part of the guide.

---

445 In what are called "intermediate frequencies" — 300 Hz to 10 MHz.
446 magdahavas.org

He shared with me his Golden Rules of Dirty Electricity mitigation, which go like this:[447]

1) Remove sources of DE first, before installing any filter.

2) Look for and fix wiring errors in the building before installing any filter.

3) If you feel worse with filters installed, remove them. If you feel way better, keep them on.

4) Filters create a strong magnetic field near them. Keep at least one foot away from your body.[448]

5) Certain sources of DE are so hard to filter out that you absolutely need to work with an expert (read on to learn what they are).

Based on Michael's advice, I've formulated my recommendations on how to reduce DE in your home as much as possible, starting as always with the cheap & easy solutions, and moving to the situations where you'll need to call an EMF expert.

447 Phone conversation with Building Biologist Michael Schwaebe, May 10th 2017.
448 electricsense.com

Dirty Electricity - Level 1

Cheap & Easy

Removing sources of DE isn't the cheapest EMF-reducing tip I'll share, but you don't have to do it all the second you put this guide down. Feel free to slowly but surely replace your DE-generating devices with better ones as your budget permits.

Get Rid Of High-DE Sources

As I shared in Chapter 1, the biggest sources of dirty electricity are converters which transform the AC electricity from your wiring into the DC current used by most electronic devices — but also any kind of electronic or electric device which works by interrupting the flow of electrical current.

The best (worst) example of a high DE-generating device is a CFL (compact fluorescent light) bulb. The way this energy-efficient light bulb saves electricity is by flickering ON and OFF at least 20,000 times per second.[449]

The same is true of most LED lights, and most fluorescent light bulbs. At the moment, I unfortunately haven't found a reliable and cheap way to verify if your particular type of lightbulb is a problem or not.

For now, my advice is to try and get rid of all these high-DE sources:

- CFL lightbulbs
- Fluorescent light bulbs
- LED light bulbs (unless tested clean)
- Halogen light bulbs (unless tested clean)
- Dimmer switches

And replace them with cleaner lightning solutions (look for my brand recommendations in a few pages):

- Incandescent, old-school light bulbs
- Incandescent halogen bulbs
- Low-DE LED bulbs

Out of all of these options, the ones I would personally recommend would be the old-school, incandescent bulbs — because they emit a kind of light that's closer to the natural light spectrum

449 Dr. Samuel Milham, Dirty Electricity: Electrification and the Diseases of Civilization.

emitted by the sun. This means this kind of light is more compatible with your body... but that's a rabbit hole we won't go into yet — maybe in a future "Non-Tinfoil" guide.

Unplug Chargers When Not In Use

I've already recommended you to tuck your laptop's charger away from your work area because it's a very high source of Magnetic Fields (MF) and Electric Fields (EF) — but these things also create dirty electricity the second they're plugged in a wall outlet, according to certified EMF specialist Eric Windheim.[450]

So simply unplug all your chargers from the wall when not in use. You'll hit 3 sources of EMFs with one stone.

450 In an interview he did with Evan Brand of the Not Just Paleo podcast.

Dirty Electricity - Level 2

Intermediate

If you're ready to invest a bit more money to reduce the levels of DE in your home, there are a few things you can do on your own.

Use DE Filters At The Main Breaker Panel

It's important to understand that there are two main reasons the electricity in your entire house can become "dirty":

1. **It comes from *inside* your home — in which case you can do something about it by getting rid of the sources.**

2. **It comes from *outside* your home.**

In the last several decades, utility companies have started dumping their extra current into the ground instead of returning it back to the station. While this saves them a bunch of money, it successfully electrifies the ground and creates stray voltage that can make your electrical system dirty.

DE generated from your neighbors' houses can also get into your home. Building Biologist Sal LaDuca explains that any house which shares the same utility transformer can transfer dirty electricity to each other.[451] Fortunately, there's a relatively easy and low-cost way to prevent this issue.

Normally, Michael Schwaebe recommends never installing DE filters unless you're 100% sure there's no wiring error in your home.[452] But there's one exception — you can safely hire an electrician to install DE filters on the receptacle right next to the main breaker panel, making sure the electricity that enters your house is as clean as possible.[453]

I highly recommend at least getting a short phone consult with a Building Biologist if you want to install dirty electricity filters near your main breaker panel, but it all comes down to putting 1 to 3 filters (don't worry, I'll share the brands below) on the outlets right next to it — often called "the receptacle". You'll have to hire an electrician for this one.

---

451 Discussion between Lloyd Burrell and Sal LaDuca, as part of ElectricSense.com's EMF Experts Solutions Club. See electricsense.com for more details.

452 If you have an EMF meter, a wiring error in your house would show up as abnormally high magnetic fields (>2 mG) in an entire room.

453 For more information, see Michael Schwaebe's presentation here: youtube.com/watch?v=ErBISqF6Afs

Measure Levels Of DE In Your House

Having a DE meter can be a great way to assess if you need to change your lighting, and whether any attempt you're making at reducing dirty electricity is working or not.

However, there's currently no recognized standard on what exactly constitutes dirty electricity, and different dirty electricity meters usually just read the Electric Field (EF) portion of DE, not giving you any information about the frequency of the current (Magnetic Fields). In plain English — it's darn complicated.

Still, if you keep those things in mind, I don't think it's a bad idea to invest in a Graham-Stetzer Microsurge Meter. Just plug it in outlets throughout your house, and you'll instantly see how dirty the electricity is.

This meter gives you a reading in Graham-Stetzer (GS) units. Ideally, you'd want to stay below 50 GS units, and probably below 25 if you're electro-sensitive.[454] Building Biologists often see readings of several hundred units to several thousands in homes or commercial buildings they visit.

454 Advice from Lloyd Burrell, EMF activist and former EHS sufferer.

Dirty Electricity - Level 3

EMF Expert

Ultimately, Dirty Electricity (DE) is a problem that's not easy to fix by yourself, and that would be better handled if you hire a certified Building Biologist to help you out.

If you find yourself in any of the following situations, then hiring a professional is the way to go:

- Your home uses solar or wind power — which are such huge sources of dirty electricity that it can literally make the occupants sick[455]
- You suffer from electro-hypersensitivity (EHS) — which means that adding filters may make your problems worse
- You don't own an EMF meter and want to make sure your house doesn't have wiring errors — in which case adding DE filters could make your problems worse
- Your house has a smart meter — a known source of DE (I'll address smart meters in a separate section)
- You live right next to a cellular tower — which can pollute surrounding homes with a ton of DE
- Your house has a variable speed swimming pool or well pump, an energy efficient HVAC system with variable speed motors or an electric car battery charger

Feel free to investigate these things on your own, but as Michael Schwaebe clearly told me during our conversation, there's no one-size-fits-all solution for the vast majority of dirty electricity problems.

455 hbelc.org

Recommended Products[456]

Our global understanding of EMF science and engineering evolves very quickly, and it is a real challenge to assess which gizmos are really worth your time and money. To get my latest endorsements and product recommendations, please visit theeemfguy.com

456 A lot of people have asked me about low-DE lighting solutions since the release of this book. This article by Building Biologist Oram Miller contains a lot of good recommendations: createhealthyhomes.com/lighting.php

Wiring Errors

Estimates will vary from one expert to another, but Building Biologist Michael Schwaebe says that about 25% of all houses where he does EMF assessments have wiring errors that create concerning levels of Magnetic Fields in the living environment.

Unfortunately, there's no real way to know if this is the case with *your* house unless you have an EMF meter and are able to measure the levels in your environment.

While most houses have Magnetic Field levels of around 1-2 mG, the levels can quickly rise up to 12 mG[457] or more when there are wiring errors present — levels linked with a dramatic increase in risks of childhood leukemia. What it can do to you, no one knows.

Here's a simple way to understand how wiring errors are created:[458]

No Wiring Error

In a normal electrical circuit, the "hot" and neutral wires are right next to each other, and their fields cancel each other.

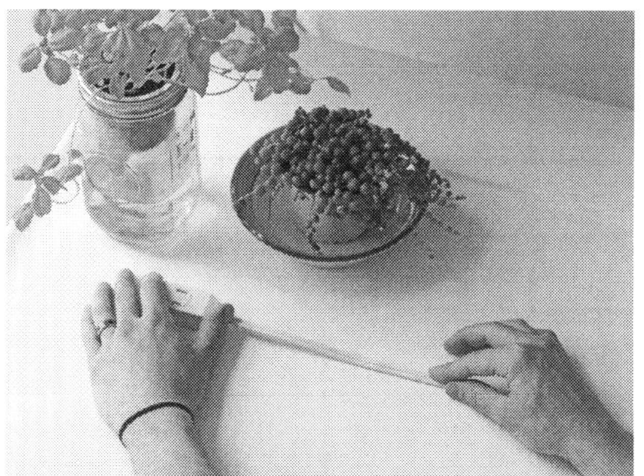

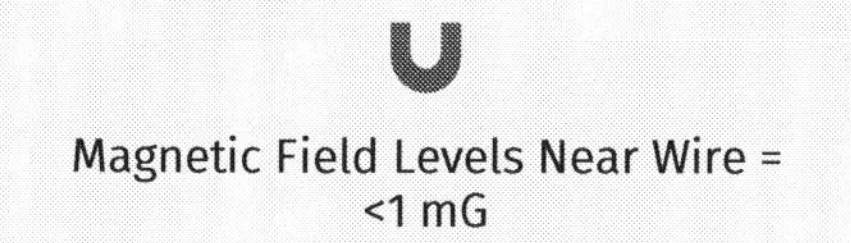

With Wiring Error

When there's a wiring error, the "hot" and neutral wires can be separated, and a big magnetic field is created in-between them.

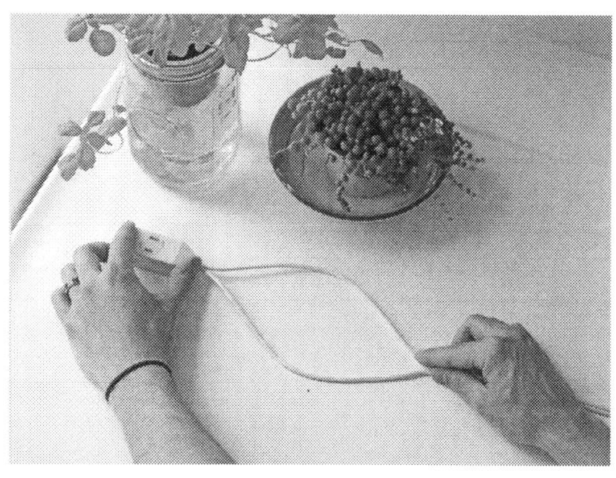

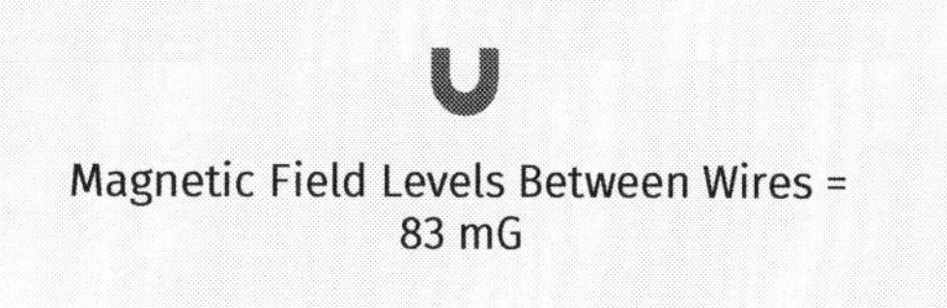

---

457 According to Building Biologist Alex Stadner from Healthy Building Science. See his website at healthybuildingscience.com/

458 Thanks to EMF consultant Michael Neuert for the inspiration. See his demonstration here:

Now, imagine that the extension cords I've used in the example above are circuits that run throughout the walls of your living room. Wiring errors can create situations where all the electricity in the wall in front of you wants to cancel all the electricity in the wall behind you — creating a giant magnetic field in the middle of the room.

The good news is that once identified, these wiring errors can be rapidly fixed by an electrician, and usually for a relatively low cost.

That being said, keep in mind that most electricians and even most electrical engineers aren't required by law to create a low-EMF electrical system in your home, and that most of them aren't even aware of the EMF problem, as explains Building Biologist Lloyd Morgan.[459]

---

youtube.com/watch?v=-M4j-YdyrVo

459 Discussion between Lloyd Burrell and Lloyd Morgan, as part of ElectricSense.com's EMF Experts Solutions Club. See electricsense.com for more details.

Current On Water Or Gas Pipes

Having unwanted current run on your water or gas pipes is another EMF problem that is hard to detect, unless you hire an EMF expert. And according to Building Biologist Frank DiCristina, this problem is present in a whopping 90% of all houses he visits when hired to do a complete EMF home assessment.[460]

This current can either come from an error in your electrical system, but also from the electricity on the water and gas pipes of your neighbors' houses getting transferred to yours.

You can easily prevent this without hiring an EMF expert: simply have a plumber install a plastic section at the water and gas main.[461] This will remove the possibility of any stray current from the ground or neighboring houses getting into your home.

---

460 Discussion between Lloyd Burrell and Frank DiCristina, as part of ElectricSense.com's EMF Experts Solutions Club. See electricsense.com for more details.

461 Consult your local plumber to see if this is allowed in your state, province and country.

Geopathic Stress

I hesitated to include this section about geopathic stress, because this EMF issue is not only pretty much ignored and unrecognized in North America... the traditional way to detect it — "dowsing" using copper, plastic or wooden rods — is also being flagged as pure pseudoscience by some scientists.[462]

But eh, millions of incredibly intelligent people still think EMFs are perfectly safe, so is that really an argument anymore?

I made the editorial choice to tell you what geopathic stress is, what it's not, and how geopathic stress experts (geomancers) recommend getting rid of it.

In my research process, I got in touch with Brian Hoyer, one of the rare EMF experts in North America who actually understands geopathic stress.

Brian first heard about Geopathic stress in his training with Dr. Klinghardt, who addresses geopathic stress with his patients in addition to other types of EMF stressors. In his search for solutions, Brian trained with Geovital Academy[463] to learn more about testing geopathic stress and clinically proven solutions.

Brian explained that geopathic stress is also known as "geoelectricity" and can be explained as naturally induced currents underground. Yes, it turns out that even "all-natural" EMFs can take a toll on your health if you're overexposed.

This geopathic stress can be generated from the interaction of the earth's magnetism with solar wind (Hartmann and Curry Lines),[464] underground water, metallic layers of the earth compressing creating a charge, and other geologic activity that gives rise to abnormally high magnetism and currents.

These disruptive natural fields can negatively impact your health when they happen deep underground, and end up changing the EMF environment at home, especially in your bedroom.

---

462 livescience.com

463 You can read more about Geovital's unique approach to EMF mitigation on their website: en.geovital.com/

464 There are many different types of geopathic grid systems that have been proposed, like the Hartmann grid — discovered in 1954 by researcher Ernst Hartmann: swissharmony.com/earth-rays/what-is-the-hartmann-grid/

In Europe, geopathic stress is generally more accepted — especially in Russia, Germany and Austria, where serious scientists have been studying the subject for decades.[465]

This is where things get a bit too woo-woo for a lot of people...

Dowsing — The Art Of Finding Hidden Things, Or Silly Superstition?

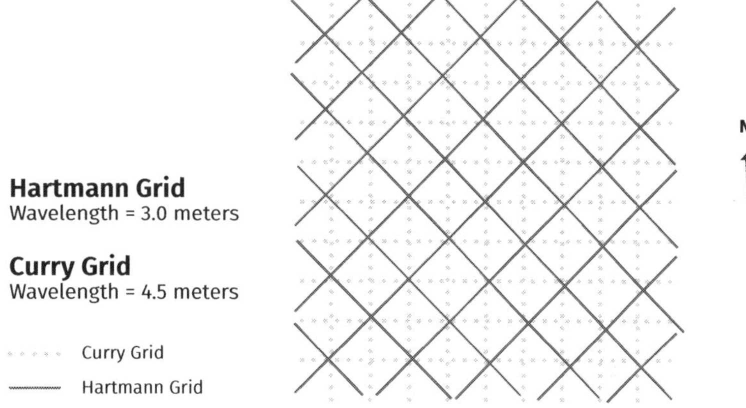

The most common way to identify geopathic stress zones is to do something called "dowsing" — an ancient practice with bizarre mechanisms that are still subject to controversy.

As paranormal researcher Stephen Wagner explains,[466] "dowsing, is the art of finding hidden things. Usually, this is accomplished with the aid of a dowsing stick, rods or a pendulum.

The dowser, by concentrating on the hidden object, is somehow able to tune in to the energy force or 'vibration' of the object which, in turn, forces the dowsing rod or stick to move. The dowsing tool may act as a kind of amplifier or antenna for tuning into the energy."

This is the slightly woo-woo, energetic kind of dowsing, which resembles applied kinesiology — more commonly known as "muscle testing".

Believe it or not, Albert Einstein himself was a dowser. In communications with a colleague in 1946[467] he said he believed that "the dowsing rod is a simple instrument which shows the reaction of the human nervous system to certain factors which are unknown to us at this time."

Then, there's a more scientific way to discover geopathic stress — using the conductive properties of copper rods. Brian Hoyer explains how it works:

"The copper rods will cross when there is energy coming up from below influencing the minerals

465 royriggs.co.uk
466 thoughtco.com
467 alberteinstein.info

in the body and causing them to be attracted to one another or pushed away. This can be demonstrated only when a person is walking over the lines in a fluid continuous motion. You can even see this easily demonstrated with an extension cord that is plugged in as you walk over it. The energy from the extension cord will cause the rods to cross or come apart as you walk over it."

Controversial or not, some open corporations like Hoffman-La Roche (one of the largest pharmaceutical companies in the world) pay dowsers a lot of money to help them find underground water streams or oil.[468]

Roche's dowser Dr. Peter Treadwell explains that "Roche uses methods that are profitable, whether they are scientifically explainable or not."

How Do I Know I'm Being Exposed To Geopathic Stress?

If you suffer from insomnia or restlessness at night, geopathic stress might be part of your problem. Here's how to tell:

1. Follow all the basic recommendations I outline in this guide (remove any wireless device from your bedroom, turn off the breakers, etc) to eliminate the common EMF offenders that are linked with poor sleep.

2. If you still can't sleep in a perfectly clean EMF environment, your next step is to sleep in another room or even just move your bed by a few feet and see how you feel. Geopathic stress zones are generally very focused (the Hartmann lines are 8 to 12 inches wide), so moving by a few feet will likely get your head out of the danger zone.

3. If you think this might be a problem, your next step is to hire an EMF consultant who understands geopathic stress and who will help you identify and mitigate the fields in your environment.

A solution for geopathic stress that Shielded Healing and Geovital professionals use are static oscillating circuits of copper wire encased in mats that are placed under the bed — which deflect geopathic stress but while still allowing the beneficial harmonics of the Schumann Resonance to come through. Of course, a thorough assessment is required to be sure that the proper strength of shielding is put in place.

I highly recommend looking for a Geovital consultant in your area.[469] You can also get in touch with

468 canadiandowsers.org
469 en.geovital.com

Brian Hoyer who generously contributed to my research by visiting his website at shieldedhealing.com

Brian has trained a team of Shielded Healing Pros. They use carefully selected professional equipment that measures the body as an antenna for RF, AC voltage, and AC current. They also test for artificial light stressors, magnetic fields, and dirty electricity. They provide solutions and proven protocols for all the problems found in homes or workplaces.

His team roams around the entire country, so if you contact him there's a good chance he might be able to visit your area soon enough for a home assessment.

Your Low-EMF Home, Room By Room

To avoid sounding like a broken record as we move forward, I'll take into consideration that you read everything I've shared about your personal EMF-emitting devices and how to handle the 6 most worrisome EMF sources in your home.

In this next part, follow me as we visit every room of a low-EMF home.

Bedroom - Level 1

Cheap & Easy

Your bedroom is the most important environment to get right — for obvious reasons. This is when your body is supposed to be in healing, resting and recharging mode.

But for most people, the opposite is happening — with more than 1 out of 4 adults in the US suffering from chronic sleep problems.[470] I cannot blame EMFs for the entire insomnia epidemic we're struck with, but I bet it's part of the equation.

Shut Down Breakers At Night

This trick doesn't cost a dime, and it takes 5 seconds to do every night. And yet, most people who simply shut down the circuit breaker to their bedroom at night report sleeping way better.

That's because all the standard 120/240V wiring in your walls emits a 6-8 foot wide Electric Field (EF) which disrupts your deep "REM" sleep and reduces your levels of melatonin. For some sensitive people, it can even trigger severe insomnia.

Remove All Devices

Make sure your smartphone is on airplane mode if you use it as an alarm clock — no worries, you'll charge it in the morning as soon as you wake up. Make sure the wifi and Bluetooth functions are turned off too, or else it will keep emitting.

If you want to be able to receive an emergency phone call, get a land line. If it's not possible, your next best bet is to set your phone as far as possible from your body during the night — ideally in a different room.

Unplug Everything

If you can't turn off the breakers at night, then make sure *not* to turn off your nightstand lamps — unplug them instead. Remember that lamps and anything electronic will radiate Electric Fields (EF) as long as they're plugged into an electrical outlet — even when turned "off".

The EF problem is even worse when the electronic device is ungrounded — and that's the case with a vast majority of lamps.

---

470 ncbi.nlm.nih.gov/books/NBK19960

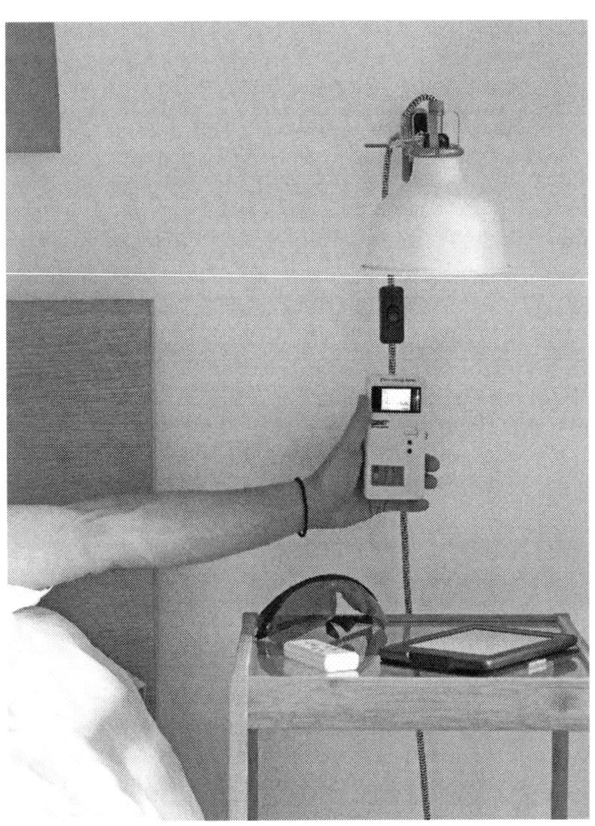

My Nightstand Lamp
Plugged In Outlet But Turned Off

EF Levels — 1" From Lamp
89 V/m

My Nightstand Lamp
Unplugged

EF Levels — 1" From Lamp
<20 V/m

EF Precautionary Safety Levels
<1.5 V/m (night)

Feel free to use a battery-powered alarm clock, but avoid electronic ones like the plague. They are a high source of both Magnetic Fields (up to 30 mG at one foot according to Martin Blank)[471] and Electric Fields.

471 Martin Blank, PhD., *Overpowered*: The Dangers of Electromagnetic Radiation (EMF) and What You Can Do about It.

Bedroom - Level 2

Intermediate

Upgrade Your Bed

The next time you change your mattress, opt for a metal-free one — for reasons that should be obvious by now.

Claus Pummer, sleep consultant and inventor of the Samina mattress, reports that people who sleep on beds containing metal can have up to 5,000 mV of EF running on their body (body voltage method). As a comparison, Building Biologists recommend staying below 10 mV at night for optimal sleep.

That being said, it's still unclear to me how much of a problem this can be if you already turn off the breakers of your bedroom at night — creating a relatively low EF environment by default.

Measure EMFs Before Using These Devices

There a couple of bedroom devices that can be a real EMF hazard, and that I wouldn't recommend using unless you have an EMF meter like mine (Cornet ED88T) and can be 100% sure they're safe.

These include:

- **CPAP Machines** — I've heard reports of those making people sick when set too close to the bed area
- **Electric Blankets** — very high source of MF, linked with miscarriages and childhood leukemia[472]
- **Electric Beds** — I've heard reports of very high levels of MF and EF from those as well

472 As reported by Daniel and Ryan DeBaun in *Radiation Nation*. microwavenews.com

Bedroom - Level 3

EMF Expert

If you hire an EMF expert or certified Building Biologist, there are 3 specific things I'd look into that could bring your low-EMF bedroom to the next level.

Grounding/Earthing

This topic is very controversial.

On one side, you have people who argue that sleeping on a grounding mat is beneficial to pretty much everyone. On the other side, you have experts demonstrating that sleeping on a grounding sheet can lead to incredibly high body voltage levels, and could do more harm than good if you don't thoroughly test how it affects your EMF exposure.

The idea behind grounding makes a lot of sense. Throughout history, mankind has always been walking barefoot on the earth (or on naturally-conductive materials such as leather) — which kept us connected to the Earth's natural magnetic field, called the "Schumann resonance".

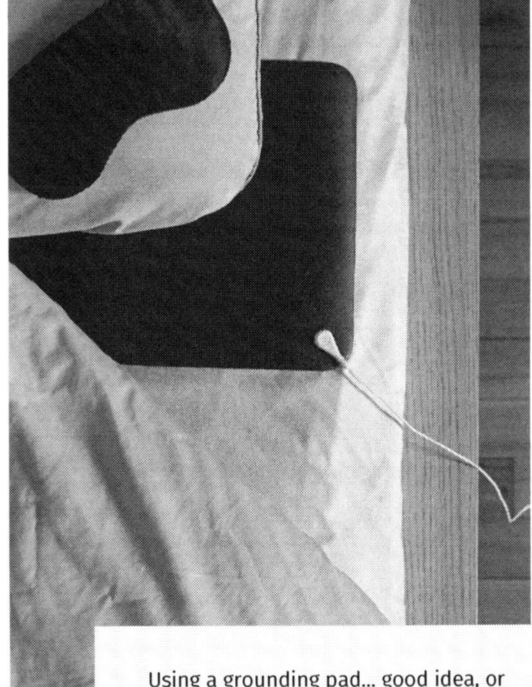

Using a grounding pad... good idea, or potential EMF disaster? It's hard to tell.

Research on Tour de France participants showed that sleeping "grounded" led to faster recovery times.[473] Other researchers like Dr. Gaetan Chevalier have studied the effects of grounding for many years and concluded that it "appears to improve sleep, normalize the day-night cortisol rhythm, reduce pain, reduce stress, shift the autonomic nervous system from sympathetic toward parasympathetic activation, increase heart rate variability, speed wound healing, and reduce blood viscosity."[474]

The more these findings see the light of the day, the more manufacturers push all sorts of

473 youtube.com
474 ncbi.nlm.nih.gov/pmc/articles/PMC4378297

grounding sheets, pads, pillows and other tools all designed to make you sleep "grounded" at night. Simply plug the pad in the ground of any electrical outlet, and you're good to go.

It all sounds good... but what happens when you use these tools in a high-EMF environment?

According to Building Biologist Eric Windheim and dozens of other EMF experts, using grounding equipment connected to an electrical outlet in a high Electric Field, high Dirty Electricity, wifi'ed environment is asking for trouble — mainly because your mat can act as a huge antenna and in fact *increase* your EMF exposure at night.

In one case, Windheim has seen a client's body voltage go up to 20,000 mV when lying on a grounding pad — that's 2,000 times the ideal levels at night.

At the moment, I do *not* recommend using any grounding equipment unless supervised by an EMF expert. Stick with the easiest, cheapest and hippiest way to ground your body — walking barefoot on the earth, in the grass or at the beach.

For an even more complete description of the different ways grounding yourself in an electrical environment can potentially do more harm than good, check out this article[475] by Building Biologist Jeromy Johnson.

475 emfanalysis.com

For EMF Geeks Only

How To Fix 95% Of The Grounding Mat Issue

If you're into DIY (do it yourself) solutions and are a real geek like me, read on.

To understand how I could safely use a grounding mat in an electrified city environment without doing more harm than good, I got in touch with Dr. Anthony G. Beck, a functional medicine practitioner who's a real expert at how changes in someone's environment can support healing.[476]

There are many potential problems with sleeping on a grounding mat that you need to be aware of:

- The mat will attract Electric Fields from the wiring in the walls and make your EF problem worse
- The mat can attract the RF signals from your wifi
- The thin wire which runs between the mat and an electrical outlet can act as an antenna too
- If the electricity in your house is dirty, it can go *up* the wire you plug into the wall outlet, and into your body
- If you connect your mat to an outside grounding rod instead of plugging it into the ground of an outlet (recommended), stray voltage present in the ground can go up the rod, up the wire, and up into your body

To fix these problems, Dr. G. Beck recommends doing the following before you sleep on a grounding mat, grounding sheets or any other indoor grounding device:

1. Shut down your bedroom's circuit breakers — eliminating most of the EF problem.

2. If possible, use a grounding rod instead of an electrical outlet. Verify that the ground isn't electrified by stray voltage, using a body voltage meter kit.

3. If you have to use an outlet, plug your mat on a Stetzerizer Dirty Electricity filter. Verify that the outlet ground is wired properly using an outlet tester.

4. Install a 100K Ohm resistor on the wire that runs between your mat and the outlet — again, to prevent dirty electricity from getting into your body.

---

476 Check out his incredible Balance Protocol Enviro which goes way more in-depth on how to heal by changing your environment at dranthonygbeck.com

5. Never use your mat during a lightning storm, which is the equivalent of standing on a golf course with a club pointed at the sky. Yikes.

Or, you can ignore all that jargon and walk barefoot in the grass or near the beach. A bit simpler.

Using A Faraday Cage/Bed Canopy

If you suffer from EHS, sleeping under an anti-EMF bed canopy can be a lifesaver.

Of course, I only recommend using those once you have completely eliminated all the usual sources of EMFs in your bedroom — and if you face external sources of EMFs coming from the outside (cell towers, smart meters, high-voltage power lines, etc.).

These canopies can cost from several hundred dollars to several thousands, and need to be properly grounded to be 100% effective. They also need to be tested by a professional to make sure they're set up properly. And you also need to shield EMF emissions coming off the floor, or else you could be creating a very problematic EMF environment.

In other words, if you're going all in and want to use such an advanced EMF mitigation technique, I highly recommend at least getting a phone consult with a Building Biologist who can advise you on how to set it up properly. It's going to be worth every penny.

Shielding, Turning Off More Breakers, And Other Shenanigans

The unfortunate truth is that even if you turn off the circuit breakers to your bedroom at night, it doesn't mean you've successfully eliminated all Electric Fields from your bedroom. After all, there could be high levels of EMFs being emitted from:

- Any wall in your bedroom that is shared with another house, apartment or condo
- The floor or ceiling or roof, if you live in a multi-story building
- Another circuit in your electrical system that happens to run in the wall right behind your pillow

The best way to know for sure that you're creating a really low-EMF environment is to hire a professional, who for example will test your body voltage as you lie down on your bed in order to find exactly *which* circuit breakers you need to turn off at night, or if there are any exterior sources of EMFs that might disrupt your sleep or make you sick.

Kitchen

High Power Kitchen Tools

Powerful electrical motors pretty much all create massive Magnetic Fields (MF). What this means to you is that you shouldn't stand right in front of these bad boys when in use:[477]

- Vitamix or other blender
- Mixer
- Dishwasher
- Toaster (I heard reports of those producing 150+ mG when in use. Toasty!)
- Electric can opener

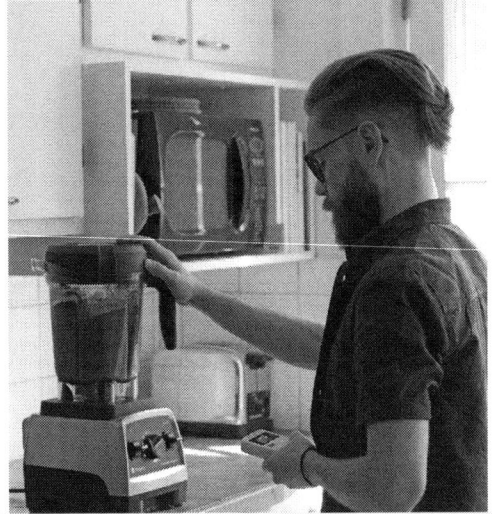

MF Levels — 1 Foot From Vitamix	MF Precautionary Safety Levels
297 mG	<1 mG (day)

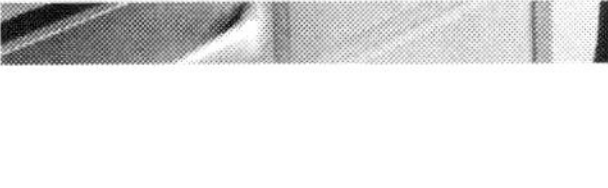

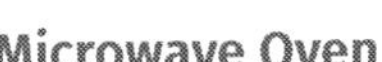

Microwave Oven

There are lot of reasons to avoid using microwave ovens, including the fact that most microwavable meals are basically a salty, MSG-sprinkled, processed mess devoid of any nutrients. From an EMF standpoint though, the problem is that all microwave ovens are known to leak considerable amounts of RF and MF radiation.

Let me be clear... they don't leak because they're defective. These devices basically come with embedded leakage.

In the US, the FDA is fine with allowing

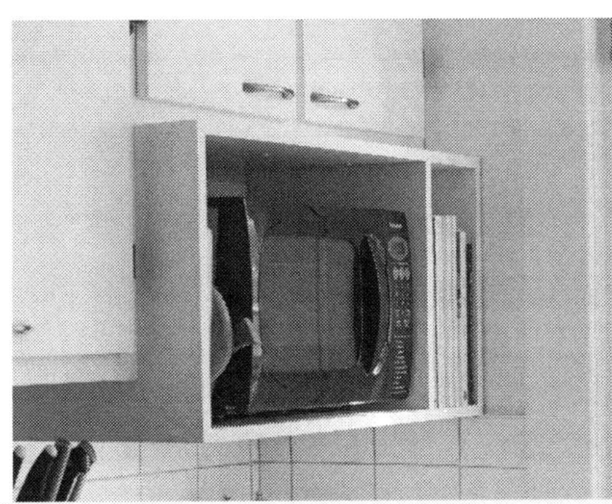

MF Levels — 1 Foot From Microwave Oven	MF Precautionary Safety Levels
41 mG	<1 mG (day)

RF Levels — 1 Foot From Microwave Oven	RF Precautionary Safety Levels
7 V/m	<0.2 V/m (day)

477 ehs.ucsd.edu

a leakage of 1 mW/cm2 in microwave (RF) radiation,[478] which amounts to a whopping 61.4 V/m — 307 times more radiation than what you should be exposed to during the day, and way more than what is emitted by multiple 4G/LTE phones.

Again — I'm not telling you to destroy your microwave oven with an axe — although I wouldn't mind if you do. But please, don't let anyone in your household stare at it while it's running.

Induction Stoves

The way an induction stove works is by creating a powerful magnetic field,[479] so it is obviously a very bad choice if you're particularly sensitive to EMFs or trying to reduce your exposure as much as possible.

In 2012, Swiss researchers found that most induction stoves exceed the already-inadequate limits set by ICNIRP when it comes to MF exposure, and expressed their concern over the fact that young children might be directly exposed at head level because of their small height.[480]

If you must use an induction stove, don't stand in front of it while you watch your food cook.

---

478 As reported by Dr. Martin Blank in *Overpowered*. See accessdata.fda.gov/scripts/cdrh/cfdocs/cfcfr/CFRSearch.cfm?CFRPart=1030&showFR=1

479 finecooking.com

480 onlinelibrary.wiley.com

Bathroom

Most devices you can use in the bathroom (hair dryers, electric razors, etc.) emit incredibly high amounts of MF. If you're particularly sensitive, you might want to reduce your use, or to try some of the tricks I'll share below to reduce your EMF exposure.

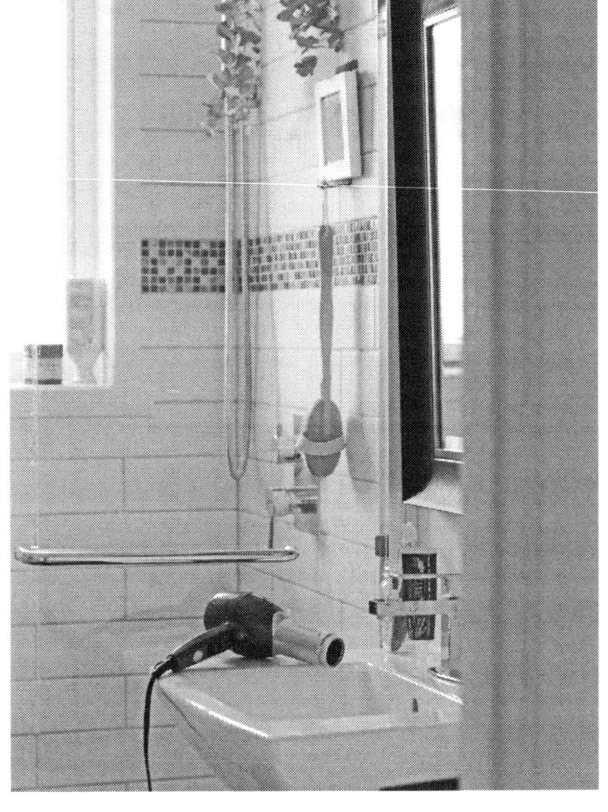

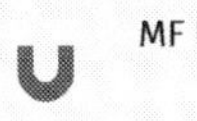

MF Levels - 6" From Hair Dryer (Hot Air) 27 mG

MF Levels - 6" From Hair Dryer (Cold Air) 4 mG

MF Precautionary Safety Levels <1 mG (day)

Hair Dryers

Hair dryers produce very large magnetic fields, which means a couple of things:

- To reduce your exposure, use a wall-mounted unit, whose motor — and magnetic fields — are far away from your head
- Use cool air over hot air. As you'll see in my test, this cuts down 99% of the radiation you're exposed to
- Avoid using an hair dryer at night — because such a high exposure could technically reduce your melatonin production
- If you're pregnant, keep that thing away from your belly while in use

Electric Razors

Martin Blank says that electric razors can emit up to 20,000 mG at 4 inches[481] — so technically they exceed even the overly generous occupational guidelines of 2,000 mG.[482]

Just use a battery-powered razor instead, and you're good to go. Rechargeable razors that you keep plugged into the wall aren't as much of a problem either.

---

481 Martin Blank, PhD., *Overpowered*: The Dangers of Electromagnetic Radiation (EMF) and What You Can Do about It.

482 pse.com

Outside Sources

A lot of people are waking up to the fact that EMFs might be a problem because they just had a smart meter installed on their house (usually without warning or consent), or because a big, scary cell tower is being installed in their neighborhood.

But ironically, they aren't aware that most of the time these outside sources of EMFs expose them to radiation levels way lower than what's emitted from their own wifi router, and orders of magnitude lower than what comes out of their smartphone 24/7.

All that being said, these outside sources of EMFs — "smart" utility meters, cellular antennas and high-voltage power lines *can* be a real hazard to your health if you spend all of your waking/sleeping hours right next to them. Here's what to look for.

Smart Meters

Around two years ago, I watched a documentary produced by Josh Del Sol called "Take Back Your Power"[483] — which explains exactly why switching your old analog electricity and gas meters for the wireless "smart" ones is a really bad idea.

There are a lot of issues around these meters, and most of them are way beyond the scope of this guide that was supposed to be relatively short but that I realize is getting pretty beefy after all.

The short version:

Everything That's Wrong With "Smart" Meters	
Privacy	"Smart" meters gather information from all your smart appliances, and transmit this information — how frequently you open the fridge, what's plugged into your walls outlets, etc. — to the utility company. Then, utility companies are allowed to sell your information to 3rd parties and make a ton of money with it.
Civil rights	When your home is connected to a "smart" meter, the utility company can shut down your power usage for any reason, at any time.

483 I highly suggest renting it for $4 on the official website: takebackyourpower.net/
484 youtube.com

Everything That's Wrong With "Smart" Meters	
Cybersecurity	Creating a "smart grid" where every household's electricity use is monitored online means that it can be hacked into. A lot of people way smarter than me when it comes to cybersecurity — including a former CIA director[484] — have said this is a really, really bad idea — for both individual households, and the regional/national Grid.
Environment	"Smart" meters need to be replaced every 5 to 7 years, compared to every 20 to 30 years for analog meters[485] — and you're the one paying the bill.
Electricity Costs	Utility companies tell everyone that installing a "smart" meter will reduce your electricity costs,[486] but a lot of people have in fact experienced a sharp rise in their monthly electricity bill.[487]
Fire Hazard	Some "smart" meters are a real fire hazard and are thought to have caused hundreds if not thousands of fires in North America alone.[488]
Dirty Electricity	"Smart" meters create a ton of dirty electricity in your house,[489] and a lot of people have reported getting sick since their installation.[490]
RF Radiation	"Smart" meters emit a strong RF signal 24/7 — which is the main issue I'll talk about... right now.

Unsurprisingly, utility companies around the world are installing "smart" meters in areas that just don't make sense — right on the other side of bedroom walls, near playgrounds, and even... in my own kitchen.

In...

My...

Kitchen...

As you can see, the "smart" meter that was installed in the apartment I'm currently renting emits a strong RF signal every 30 seconds which blasts me with peaks of 5.24 V/m while I prepare dinner next to it.

485 smartgridawareness.org
486 thestar.com
487 emfsafetynetwork.org
488 emfsafetynetwork.org
489 See the proof here: youtube.com/watch?time_continue=1&v=4NTSejgsjTc
490 mainecoalitiontostopsmartmeters.org

Now, this is the perfect example of what any sane person would call a very stupid use of modern technology. Why would you use a signal so strong? Why would you install it in a freaking kitchen, near sleeping areas, or expose children? And why do they need to transmit data every 30 seconds instead of once a day?

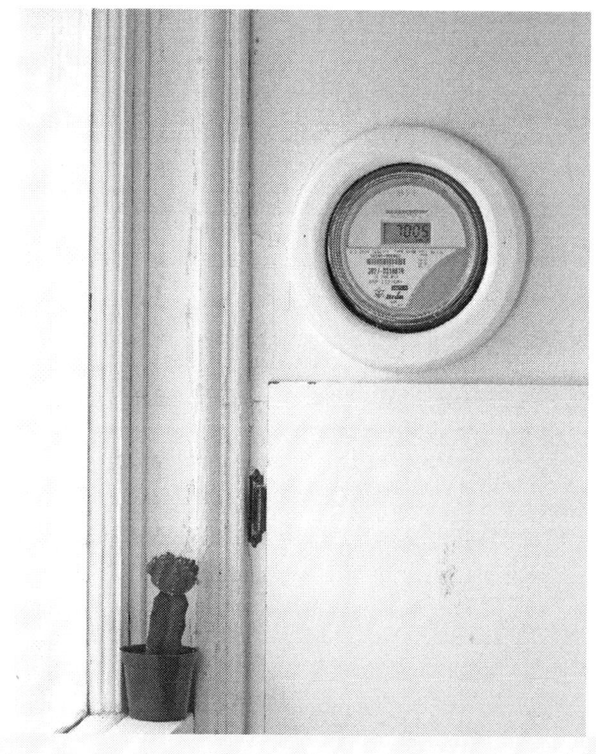

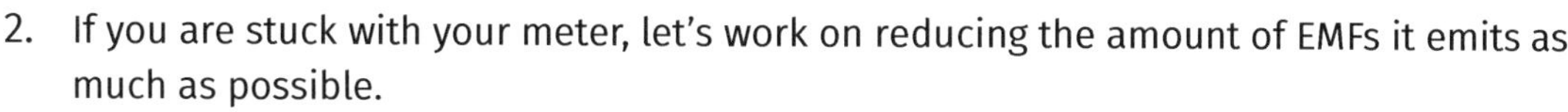

RF Levels - 1 Foot From Smart Meter 5.24 V/m

RF Precautionary Safety Levels <0.2 V/m (day)

Don't answer. These are all rhetorical questions.

I'm here to talk about solutions, so let's see what you can do about the issue:

1. Ask your utility company to opt-out of the "smart" meter program, and to replace your "smart" meter with an old-school, analog one instead.

   Depending on where you live, the utility company might charge you a monthly penalty, do it for free, or just say "no" in certain states or cities where they have the right to do so.

2. If you are stuck with your meter, let's work on reducing the amount of EMFs it emits as much as possible.

   So first, do the best you can to reduce the amounts of dirty electricity in your home — following the recommendations I've made sooner. Then, think about shielding.

   You can install a Smart Meter Guard on it, which will probably cut down the radiation a lot — but understand that if you remove 100% of the radiation, the utility might not receive your consumption data and knock on your door to verify what's wrong with your meter.

   You can also do like I did and put tinfoil on top of the meter as a short-term solution — which in my case cut down the EMF emissions at 1 foot by a whopping 73% (1.44 V/m peaks).

3. Hire a certified Building Biologist or EMF expert to help you measure the levels you're exposed to, and properly shield your meter.

   In reality, without a proper EMF meter you'll always be unable to tell:

- If your particular model of "smart" meter emits every 6 seconds, every minute, or once a day
- How much EMF radiation it's emitting — certain models have been found to emit more RF radiation than 100 cell phones[491]
- If the homemade shielding solution you're using is doing its job and reducing the signals getting into your house
- If your own meter is a real problem, or if the neighbors' meters are a biggest problem

Everything on this section applies to electricity "smart" meters, "smart" gas meters, "smart" water meters, and any other digital meter that's installed on your home.

491 As confirmed by Building Biologist Oram Miller and multiple EMF activists. See youtube.com/watch?v=a6-hcOr-sxA

"The demand is increasing. We need to fill the constant demand for faster data transfers, better coverage." This is your fault, just as much as it is mine. We users are begging for the Telecom companies to install more and more cell towers, and pack them with dozens of antennas.

The problem is that this exponential growth for cellular networks is done with basically useless safety standards, and with an industry that's 0% liable about possible health effects — at least in the US, thanks to the 1996 Telecom Act.

The result is that people like you and me live in cities where there are up to dozens of cell towers in a single square mile.

The problem is that there's solid evidence that living even as far as 1,500 feet (500m) from a cell tower can harm your health in a significant way.

Distance From Cell Tower	Symptoms[492]
<500m	Increased cancer risks
<400m	Sleep disturbance, tiredness, depressive mood, triple the cancer risks
<300m	Tiredness
<200m	Headaches, sleep disturbance, discomfort
<100m	Irritability, depression, loss of memory, dizziness, libido decrease

What's the safe distance? Most experts I've studied seem to think that a distance of at least 400 meters between a cell tower and your house is smart.

Sounds good Nick, but how do I know if there are cell towers and antennas near my house if I'm in the middle of a crowded city? Am I being blasted as I'm reading these lines? Don't panic just yet.

492 Based on these studies: ncbi.nlm.nih.gov/pubmed/12168254, powerwatch.org.uk/news/20050722_bamberg.asp, sciencedirect.com/science/article/pii/S0048969711005754 and powerwatch.org.uk/news/20041118_naila.pdf

Here's what you need to do to address the cell tower problem. Ask yourself the following questions, in the following order:

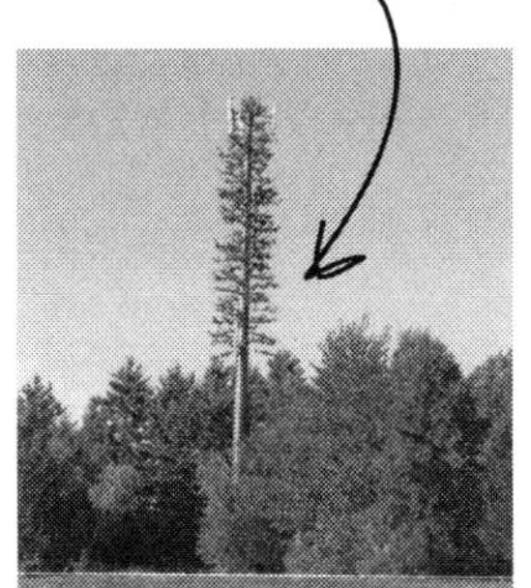

1. Is there a cell tower that you can clearly see from one of your house or apartment windows? Is there a cellular antenna on the roof of your building?[493]

   If so, I highly suggest hiring a certified Building Biologist to take measurements in your environment, or at least renting an EMF meter (like the Acousticom 2) to verify how much of this radiation is getting inside your home.

   Depending on the type of cell antenna you're dealing with, its power, its technology and a bunch of other factors — you might just find that this tower is no issue, at least for now. With the exponential increase in our EMF environment, I suggest re-testing every 6 months to make sure it's still true.

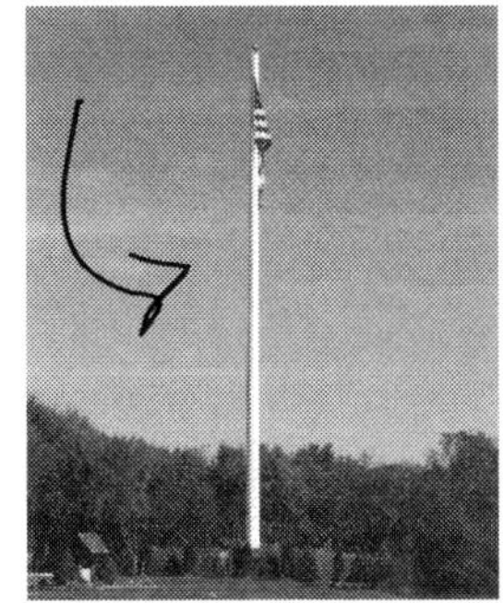

2. Are you dealing with hidden cell antennas? Believe it or not, there's an antenna hidden in every single one of the pictures on this page.

   Yeah, "kind of messed up" are the words that come to mind here. Cell antennas are getting harder and harder to detect, and very soon there are going to be 120,000 antennas in traffic light signs in New York City alone.[494]

   There is a great website — AntennaSearch.com — which can help you find all the cell towers in your area — but please note that the website is only available in the US.

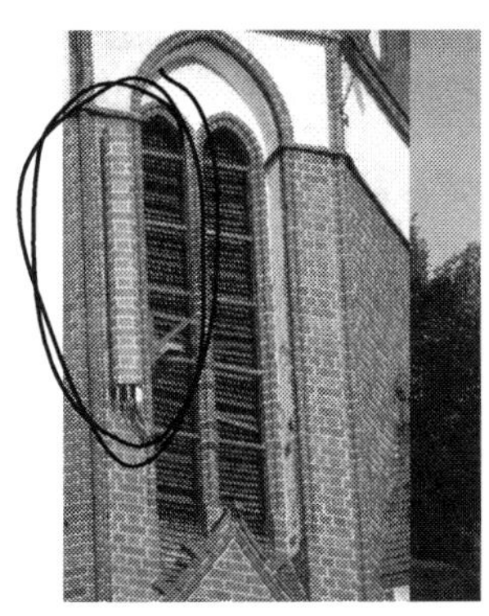

3. The unfortunate truth is... as Building Biologist Peter Sierck explains,[495] you can't really tell if you're being overexposed to RF radiation because of a cell tower nearby, unless you invest in a

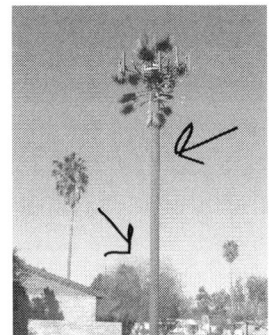

---

493 With building owners being paid up to several thousand bucks a month to set up a "completely harmless" cellular tower on their rooftop, this problem is spreading like wildfire. electrosmogprevention.org

494 forbes.com

495 Discussion between Lloyd Burrell and Peter Sierck, as part of ElectricSensecom's EMF Experts Solutions Club. More details at electricsense.com/.

meter,[496] or hire a professional.

4. If you end up finding out that a cell tower is literally blasting away at your pillow through your bedroom's window — it doesn't necessarily mean you'll have to pack your stuff in a hurry and get the hell out.

   There are many ways to shield your home or apartment from exterior signals, but never attempt any kind of shielding unless you can take measurements before and after your intervention. If you screw it up, you could in fact *increase* the radiation you're exposed to.

High-Voltage Power Lines

Everything I mentioned about cell towers still applies here. The difference is that high-voltage power lines generate powerful Magnetic Fields (MF), not RF radiation — and that MF cannot be easily shielded.

Exposure to low level magnetic fields has been linked with increases in childhood leukemia.[497] The possible effects on adults are very unclear, but the advocacy group Powerwatch UK reports that after compiling more than 300 studies on power lines and low levels of MF, more than 200 of them found negative health effects.[498]

So... how close is too close? Let's look at the consequences reported at different distances:

Distance From High-Voltage Power Line	Effect
<300m	Exposing children doubles their risk of developing an immune system disorder later in life[499]
<100m	Increased risk of brain cancer (meningioma)[500]
<61m[501]	Doubling in risks of poor sperm motility or morphology[502]
<50m	Doubling in risks of Alzheimer's after 10 years[503]

Of course, different types of power lines emit different amounts of MF. The strongest types of power lines (400kV) typically produce less than 0.5 mG at 200 meters,[499] so that's probably what

496 For $179, the Cornet ED88T would be your cheapest solution, if you want to be in charge and measure 3 different kinds of EMFs in your environment.
497 Most studies show increases in childhood leukemia at MF levels over 2 mG, which is why I stick with the precautionary levels of 1 mG during the day.
498 powerwatch.org.uk
499 ncbi.nlm.nih.gov/pubmed/17543004

you could say is a "safe distance" to have between your house and the source.

Again, you can never be 100% sure of whether the power lines outside your home are too close, or virtually harmless — unless you're armed with an EMF-meter.

It's really hard to tell which type of power line you're dealing with just by looking at it, and in some cases regular power lines on your street might be a bigger problem if they are very close to your sleeping area.

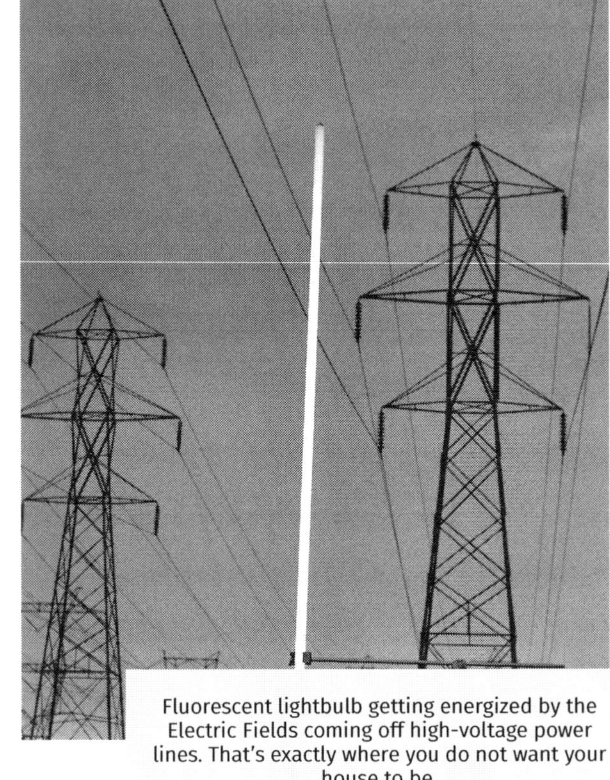

Fluorescent lightbulb getting energized by the Electric Fields coming off high-voltage power lines. That's exactly where you do not want your house to be.

500 ncbi.nlm.nih.gov/pubmed/21792884
501 The typical levels of exposure 61 m from a high-voltage power line are 1.8 mG. See niehs.nih.gov/health/topics/agents/emf
502 ncbi.nlm.nih.gov/pubmed/21792884
503 ncbi.nlm.nih.gov/pubmed/18990717
504 emwatch.com

Children

Being Exposed Since Day 1

TTT
The Three Things

1. Shield Your Body During Pregnancy
2. Put Devices On Airplane Mode Around Children Of Any Age — Especially At Night
3. Preach By Example & Disconnect, Together With Your Family

Let's End On A Depressing Note, Shall We?

I must admit... it's really hard for me to keep my cool while writing this part. Because the fact is that those who will suffer the most from our current (unknowingly) stupid use of technology are children — and the next generations to come.

To avoid sounding like a broken record, I won't repeat everything I've recommended you should do in the *Personal Devices* and *Home* sections. If you do just the top 3 things in these sections, you'll already eliminate 90% of the risks associated with EMFs your children could have faced.

Keep in mind that anything I've shared so far in this guide affects children in an exponential way, because a child's body contains more water which makes it absorb way more radiation — in a 1-year-old, twice as much as in an adult.[505]

But I do realize that the biggest challenge all parents are facing these days is: how do you get your children to change the way they use technology in a world where iPads have replaced teddy bears?

When I make bold statements like these, a lot of young adults around my age (I just turned 30) tell me I'm overstating the issue. But what they don't realize is how much our world has changed in the last 30 years...

505 As reported by Daniel and Ryan DeBaun in *Radiation Nation*. See https://webarchive.nationalarchives.gov.uk/20100910163012/http://www.iegmp.org.uk/documents/iegmp_6.pdf

Born With Technology

Age -1 — It's Going To Be A Bumpy Ride...

In 1987, little Nicolas Pineault was born in an environment with no wifi, cell phone antenna or any of that stuff. But 30 years later in 2017, children are born in an environment where there are signals *everywhere*.

It's hard being a fetus these days. If the egg and spermatozoid both survive the intensive lap zapping most parents put their reproductive organs through (thanks, Macbook Pro!), you just pray to the universe that you don't start your journey in this world with serious DNA damage.

No, the game isn't won the second you finally become a 100-celled embryo around the 3rd week. There's still so much to do — and you'll have to develop 250,000 neurons every minute for the next 8 months.[506] And somehow people think all you do is sleep?

Hopefully, mom doesn't start blasting you with strong cell phone signals right next to her belly. In one study, pregnant physiotherapists who used a medical device emitting RF radiation for just a couple seconds every day saw their risks of miscarriage increase by 3-fold[507] (true, the levels were higher than what a 4G phone emits).

If mom spends a ton of time in a high-EMF environment or uses her laptop on her lap, I know she's going to protect you with a Belly Blanket or Belly Band which are very effective ways to shield your developing body against cell phones and wifi.

She'll also make sure she sleeps in a low-EMF environment, following each of Nicolas Pineault's very wise recommendations she's read in this guide — to the best of her abilities. Who knows, she might even hire a Building Biologist[508] in order to be 100% sure that her home is safe.

We're almost there. Brace yourself, because the bigger you get, the less protected you'll be from the outside environment — and the more RF signals you'll get exposed to.

506 ncbi.nlm.nih.gov/books/NBK234146
507 ncbi.nlm.nih.gov/pmc/articles/PMC1469943
508 To find a Building Biologist in your area, visit hbelc.org/find-an-expert

Age 0 — You've Made It!

You've made it, but don't celebrate too much just yet. You're soon going to meet your nemesis — the evil baby monitor — that mom has no idea can be a source of RF radiation way worse than a 4G cell phone.

As she gets informed, mom is going to opt for safer solutions to make sure you're OK:[509]

- A D-Link ethernet enabled camera
- For European parents, the NUK BabyPhone (Only available in Europe)
- For American parents, the SmartNOVA Baby Monitor

Your head is way smaller than the large head of big S.A.M. from Chapter 3, which means that having a cell phone next to your head to tell grandma your first words is out of the question. Devices must always be in airplane mode around you.

Get smart, and use your cute eyes trick... it might just persuade your parents to buy a nice EMF-blocking hat.

Age 1 — Meet Your New Nanny

There's a new member in the family that's going to take care of you, and that Parents Magazine has wisely called the "perfect babysitter"[510] — the latest iPad.

Hopefully your parents tell the "nanny" to always stay on airplane mode while she's teaching you what the world is all about, or else the RF signal will get through your eyes and into your brain from just looking at it.[511]

But yeah, the peer pressure is already on. At that point, 44% of your age 1 friends also play games on an iPad or smartphone every single day.[512]

---

509 See emfanalysis.com/safe-baby-monitor/ for additional recommendations from Building Biologist Jeromy Johnson.

510 As reported by researcher and EMF activist Devra Davis, PhD.

511 As reported by Devra Davis, PhD. See ieeexplore.ieee.org/document/7369205/metrics

512 The stats I'm reporting are no joke, and date back from 2013. The real numbers are probably way higher at the time of this writing. aap.org

Age 2 — You Know The Deal

You're getting bigger, and there's a 28% chance you don't even need help to navigate around on any device. iPad, iPhone, laptops... old news — you can't wait for the next gadget to come out, and you've been discussing the latest OS developments with your teddy bear. There's even a 13% chance that your parents will allow you to purchase your own apps![513]

You're even starting to do your potty training using the famous iPotty. Never let your little sister play with your iPad while you do your thing!

Age 4 — You're The One In Charge Now

Look, you've been using a smartphone for years... isn't it about time you get your own?

Good news, because it turns out that at your age, there's a 75% chance you'll own a smartphone, and a 50% chance you'll even have your own TV — even if you happen to live in an urban, low-income, minority community!

Age 6 — They Have Free Wifi!

School can get boring at times, but don't worry — at least the wifi is free.

If you get lucky, you'll even be in one of the many classrooms where everyone gets their own iPad! Unfortunately, this exposes you to massive doses of wifi signals... but eh, how bad can it really be? Everyone is doing it.

If they get too worried, Mom and dad can consult the Environmental Health Trust website to learn more about how to make schools aware of the EMF problem — and maybe have them install a simple switch to turn the wifi off when not in use, like a Finnish school did in 2017.[514]

Age 7 — Are You An Addict?

Seriously... can't you leave your iPhone just for a bit... play outside, do something? Or are you like 10% of all children in South Korea who are so addicted to the Internet they need to spend time in digital rehab camps?[515]

---

513 As reported by EMF scientist Devra Davis, PhD.
514 ehtrust.org
515 abc.net.au

Age 11 — The Internet Never Sleeps

It's hard to sleep when there are so many cool things to do, and so many social media updates happening in real time!

At this age, you fall in a category where 10% of your friends check their phones at least 10 times during the night to make sure they never miss a notification.[516]

Age 12 — Anxious Yet?

This online world might be getting on your nerves a bit. In the last 5 years alone, the risk of people your age calling for help because of serious anxiety has risen by 42%.[517]

Can we blame it on the selfie culture? On the EMFs? On something else? No one really knows.

Age 14 — You Basically Live On Your Cell Phone

If you've been talking on a cell phone for more than 4 years like most of your friends, you've unfortunately increased your risks of developing brain cancer by 4-fold.[518] There's a steady rise in cancers in teenagers,[519] so that's a bit concerning.

But even if you had this kind of information it's really hard to get off the phone, and there's a 50% chance you would consider yourself "literally addicted" to it.[520] Just like 27% of parents who report being addicted too, and preach by example.

Your smartphone is part of your life, and you carry it around in your pocket all the time. You spend around 9 hours a day on your phone or other device.[521]

There's also a 75% chance you put it right underneath your pillow as you sleep.[522] Maybe it's one of the reasons 65% of teens your age take 30 minutes or more to fall asleep, and that 23% of them suffer from insomnia?[523]

---

516 bbc.com
517 telegraph.co.uk
518 ehtrust.org
519 journals.plus.org
520 cnn.com
521 forbes.com
522 ehtrust.org
523 ncbi.nlm.nih.gov/pubmed/23611716

Age 16 — They Expect You To Do *What*?

Get off your phone. Have responsibilities. Live in the real world for once. Put that thing on airplane mode at night...

What's the deal with all these new restrictions? You just don't get it. Your parents are probably just control freaks.

At least they aren't anti-technology like Bill Gates[524] and Steve Jobs[525] — or else they would have forbidden you from ever using a cell phone before age 14.

524 bgr.com
525 nytimes.com

The Point

Education about how to use technology in a safer, more humane way, where you don't forget there's a real world out there, starts in the womb.

If you have children who are addicted to their cell phones: instead of trying to take away what they consider to be a fundamental human right — being online 24/7 — educate them.

Stress the importance of getting your fix of nature, create device-free zones and digital detox weekends — and let your children see what it feels like to re-connect with real life once in awhile.

And if the need be, bribe your teens to make them put their phone on airplane mode at night. They'll notice how better they sleep, and eventually come to the obvious conclusion that there might just be something to this EMF thing.

Summary - How To Protect Children From EMFs

Put Devices On Airplane Mode	Turn Off Breakers To Every Bedroom At Night	Setup Your Wifi Router Far From Living Areas
Ditch Baby Monitors And DECT Phones	Shield Yourself During Pregnancy	Preach By Example & Disconnect
Turn Off The Wifi At Night	Tuck Away Cords & Chargers	Get Your Home Inspected By A Building Biologist

Recommended Products

Our global understanding of EMF science and engineering evolves very quickly, and it is a real challenge to assess which gizmos are really worth your time and money. To get my latest endorsements and product recommendations, please visit theeemfguy.com.

Conclusion

ALL THAT BEING SAID

Are We Doomed?

YOU Are In Control

How Can I Help?

Are We Doomed?

It's 11:07pm. In a hipsterish-looking bar in Montreal, I'm sharing a nice pint of cider with a friend I haven't seen in ages.

An all-too-common buzzing sound interrupts our conversation. My friend reaches out to his front pocket, pulls out his iPhone 7, and quickly reads his notifications. It's a text from his wife 6 months pregnant with his first child, wishing him good night — and sending a bunch of kisses.

Quick 2-thumbed reply. Phone goes back in pocket. Quick apology. I smile and wave my hand to let him know it's fine, but at the same time I feel a profound malaise...

Is this really the right time? Should I give my friend the very-unsolicited advice to put his phone on Airplane Mode if he plans on having a second child, or if he just cares about the health of his Johnson?

I already know how the conversation will go.

I'll do my best to tell him in a very relaxed tone — the kind of tone you'd use to chit-chat about the weather while waiting uncomfortably in a packed elevator. But then he'll ask the obvious question... "Why?" — and then I'll do my best to give him the very short version of what you learned in this guide, without monopolizing the next 4 hours of his life.

And soon enough, I'll see my friend starting to look around, noticing the dozens of smartphones set on the other patrons' tables, picturing invisible radiation coming off each one of them, and starting to shift uncomfortably in his chair. Thanks, Nick.

He'll be probably feel the exact way you're probably feeling right now after having read this guide — a bizarre mix of shock, fear, disgust, urgency and hopefully a bit of relief that you at least know now the truth about how stupid our current use of technology is, and what you should do about it.

The worst part is how crushingly powerless he'll probably feel while adding "EMFs" to the laundry list of concerns we're all constantly bombarded with these days — wars, politics, terrorism, GMOs, toxic chemicals, global pollution, and inequalities of all kinds.

At this point, I'll see that he's clearly had enough doom and gloom for today — and won't even talk about the fact that things will likely get way worse in the next few years.

I won't even tell him that while the imminent rollout of the next-generation 5G cellular network will enable incredible technological advances like self-driving cars,[526] smart cities filled with billions of sensors forming what's called "The Internet Of Things" (IoT)[527] and make clean energy cheaper than coal[528] — it's also going to increase the levels of EMF radiation we're exposed to by orders of magnitude.[529]

I won't tell him that while users will be busy enjoying the incredible download speeds 5G will bring to the table (up to 50X faster than the current 4G/LTE), and while the industry will make trillions in profits, 5G technology will also require installing millions of new cellular antennas — possibly one at every street corner,[530] and on most traffic light poles.[531]

And I won't even tell him that most people working for any industry closely benefiting from a quick rollout of 5G will likely send me hate mail for having the insolence to "slow down human progress", and accuse me of being a quack — staying completely blind even when faced with the almost-overwhelming scientific evidence showing that non-ionizing radiation is making people sick.

No, I won't tell him that. Instead I'll give him the good news and end on a good note...

YOU Are In Control

You can sit around and wait for the Government to fix things. But our institutions are not only often in a position serious conflicts of interest when it comes to EMFs... they'll also get such a huge paycheck in taxes when the 5G technology rolls out that they'll probably take action as fast as they did for trans fats, banning the heart attack-inducing substance around 60 years after its introduction.

You can wait for corporations to change their current technologies for safe ones. *Yes*, they should be the ones held accountable! But the harsh reality is that all they're doing is playing by the rules of our broken safety guidelines, and that they have exactly zero reasons to invest the billions in R&D which will likely be required to develop safer wireless devices.

Or, now that you're aware of the problem, you can start asking for safe technologies. You can post on Apple and Samsung's Facebook wall, telling them you want phones that emit way less radiation

526 computerworlduk.com
527 businessinsider.com
528 technologyreview.com
529 draxe.com
530 cio.com
531 mobile.nytimes.com

— and link to this YouTube presentation by Dr. Martin Pall while you're at it.[532] You can talk about this guide to 10 people you know, and empower them to talk to 10 other people — helping create such a high consumer demand that one visionary corporation will decide to disrupt the entire Telecom industry and launch a safer cell phone.

With awareness and education comes incredible power. Once the first "healthier" smartphone hits the market, do you really know anyone who's not going to want it? And how do you think this is going to affect sales of the old, now clearly "unsafe" phones?

If you're the engineer type, you might even be the one who invents a next-generation of healthier wireless signals — maybe one that would be unpolarized,[533] that would have a different modulation, a different pulsing, that would use frequencies, or run on scalar energy... who knows! This is all over my head too — but this is research that needs to be done.

Think this is all utopia? Just look at what happened with organic foods, or what happened with the gluten-free movement in the last decade alone. Both of these multi-billion industries were built from the ground up because of high consumer awareness sparked by grassroots movements.

In a few decades from now, historians might just consider the early 2000's the medieval times of modern technology, and wonder how on Earth were people not aware they were zapping their cells with such primitive devices. How silly.

No, we're not doomed. We're just victims of a society where profits have been put first, and safety second — and where most people think that the fact you can legally buy something automatically makes it safe.

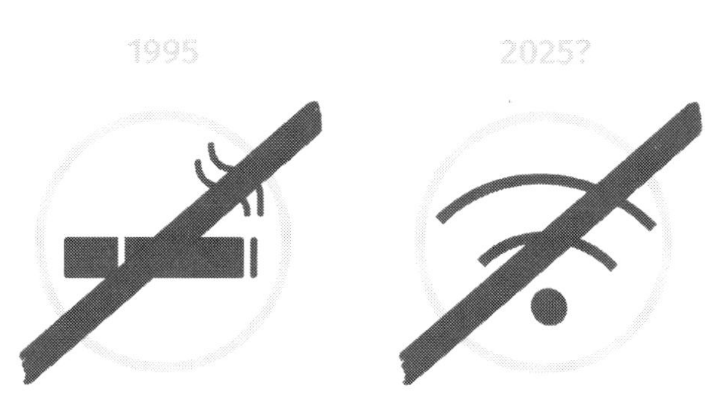

Take a deep breath, put your phone on Airplane Mode, and reconnect with nature. We'll all need a clear head, an open mind and a positive attitude to get through this.

---

532 This one always makes skeptics run away in fear: m.youtube.com/watch?v=Pjt0iJThPU0

533 In 2015 Panagopoulos et al. theorized that the main reason man-made non-ionizing radiation affects our cells' calcium channels so much at such low levels is that these EMFs are polarized, while most natural EMFS (like sunlight) are unpolarized. See ncbi.nlm.nih.gov/pmc/articles/PMC4601073/

How Can I Help?

If this guide has made a difference in your life, I would definitely be grateful if you spread the word about it.

Grab a copy for your friends, family members, coworkers... or even send one to your mayor, or State legislator!

Our online publishing company N&G Média inc. gives a percentage of its profits to nonprofit groups that are working hard to spread the word about the EMF issue and make a real change in the world, and I invite you to do the same.

I highly recommend supporting the amazing work of the Environmental Health Trust which is one of the most important non-profit organizations fighting to make real change happen.

Since I first published this book in late 2017, I've been spending all of my time sharing more EMF-related information, and most of it is free. To get my latest updates and hear about the new exciting solutions I'm working on to try and fix the EMF problem please visit https://theemfguy.com/

ANNEXES

Complete References

Annexes

(Visit nontinfoilemf.com/sources for the full links)

Annex 1

Chapter 4 — Can EMFs Affect Sleep?

Table 1

Studies	RF Radiation (V/m)	Effect	Study	Source
A	0.047-0.22	Fatigue, depressive tendency, sleeping disorders, concentration difficulties, cardio- vascular problems reported with exposure to GSM 900/1800 MHz cell phone signal at base station level exposures.	Oberfeld, 2004	vws.org
B	0.14	In adults (30-60 yrs) chronic exposure caused sleep disturbances, (but not significantly increased across the entire population).	Mohler et al., 2010	ncbi.nlm.nih.bov
C	0.19-0.64	RFR from cell towers caused fatigue, headaches, sleeping problems.	Navarro et al., 2003	emf-portal.org
D	0.19-0.43	Adults (18-91 yrs) with short-term exposure to GSM cell phone radiation reported headache, neurological problems, sleep and concentration problems.	Hutter et al., 2006	ncbi.nlm.nih.gov
E	0.43-0.61	RFR related to headache, concentration and sleeping problems, fatigue.	Kundi, 2009	emf-portal.org
F	13.72	An 18% reduction in REM sleep (important to memory and learning functions).	Mann and Roschke, 1996	emf-portal.org

Table 2

Studies	RF Radiation (SAR W/kg)	Effect	Study	Source
G	0.25	Delayed REM sleep in rats.	Mohammed et al., 2013	sciencedirect.com
H	1	Impaired sleep.	Huber et al., 2003	ncbi.nlm.nih.bov

Studies	RF Radiation (SAR W/kg)	Effect	Study	Source
I	1	GSM cell phone use modulates brain wave oscillations and sleep EEG.	Huber et al., 2003	ncbi.nlm.nih.gov
J	1	Cell phone RFR during waking hours affects brain wave activity. (EEG patterns) during subsequent sleep.	Achermann et al., 2000	emf-portal.org
K	1	Sleep patterns and brain wave activity are changed with 900 MHz cell phone radiation exposure during sleep.	Borbely et al., 1999	emf-portal.org
L	1.95	Reduction in deep sleep.	Lowden et al., 2011	emf-portal.org
M	2	Pulse-modulated RFR and MF affect brain physiology (sleep study).	Schmid et al., 2012	ncbi.nlm.nih.gov

Annex 2

Chapter 5 — Can EMFs Affect Brain Cancer Risks?

Findings	Study	Source
Increased risk of brain tumors, especially on the same side	Bortkiewicz et al., 2017	ncbi.nlm.nih.gov
Increased risk of brain tumors	Myung et al., 2009	ncbi.nlm.nih.gov
Increased risk of brain tumours especially in long-term users (≥10 years)	Prasad et al., 2017	ncbi.nlm.nih.gov
Increased risks of glioma	Carlberg and Hardell, 2012	ncbi.nlm.nih.gov
Possible association between heavy mobile phone use and brain tumours	Coureau et al., 2014	ncbi.nlm.nih.gov
Occupational magnetic field exposure increases the risk of glioblastoma	Villeneuve et al., 2002	ncbi.nlm.nih.gov
Glioma and acoustic neuroma should be considered to be caused by EMF emissions from cell phones	Carlberg and Hardell, 2013	ncbi.nlm.nih.gov
Mobile phone radiation causes brain tumors and should be classified as a probable human carcinogen (Class 2A)	Morgan et al., 2015	ncbi.nlm.nih.gov

Annex 3

Chapter 5 — Can EMFs Affect Breast Cancer Risks?

Findings	Study	Source
Increased risk of breast cancer in radio operators	Tynes et al., 1996	ncbi.nlm.nih.gov
Women under 50 were 7X more likely to develop oestrogen receptor-positive breast cancer when exposed to magnetic field levels over 1 mG	Feychting et al., 1998	ncbi.nlm.nih.gov
Plausible link between EMF and breast cancer	Caplan et al., 2000	ncbi.nlm.nih.gov
Occupational exposure to magnetic fields over 25 mG increases risks of breast cancer by 3-fold	Carlberg and Hardell, 2012	ncbi.nlm.nih.gov
Cluster of male breast cancer in office workers exposed to high levels of magnetic fields	Milham, 2004	ncbi.nlm.nih.gov
Long-term significant occupational exposure to ELF MF may certainly increase the risk of both Alzheimer's disease and breast cancer	Davanipour and Sobel, 2009	ncbi.nlm.nih.gov
Possible link between magnetic fields exposure and breast cancer	Chen et al., 2013	ncbi.nlm.nih.gov
EMF exposure may be associated with the increase risk of male breast cancer	Sun et al., 2013	ncbi.nlm.nih.gov
Low levels of magnetic fields increase risks of breast cancer	Zhao et al., 2014	emf-portal.org

Annex 4

Chapter 5 — Can EMFs Affect Men's Fertility?

Table 1

Studies	RF Radiation (V/m)	Effect	Study	Source
A	0.036	Reduced sperm count in mice.	Behari and Kesari, 2006	J. Behari and K. K. Kesari, "*Effects of Microwave Radiations on Reproductive System of Male Rats*," Embryo Talk, 1, 2006, pp. 81-85 (cannot be found online)
B	0.5-0.6	Sperm morphology abnormalities in mice.	Otitoloju et al., 2010	ncbi.nlm.nih.gov

Studies	RF Radiation (V/m)	Effect	Study	Source
C	0.79-2	Irreversible infertility in mice.	Magras and Zenos, 1997	ncbi.nlm.nih.gov
D	1.37	Significant degeneration of seminiferous epithelium in mice at 2.45 GHz, 30-40 min.	Saunders and Kowalczuk, 1981	ncbi.nlm.nih.gov
E	1.37-1.94	Laptop using wifi for 4 hours. Significant decrease in progressive sperm motility and an increase in sperm DNA fragmentation.	Avendano et al., 2012	ncbi.nlm.nih.gov
F	43.41	A 24.6% drop in testosterone and 23.2% drop in insulin after 12 hrs of pulsed RFR exposure.	Navakatikian, 1994	In "*Biological Effects of Electric and Magnetic Fields, Volume 1*" D.O. Carpenter (ed) Academic Press, San Diego, CA, 1994, pp. 333-342. 1994

Table 2

Studies	RF Radiation (SAR W/kg)	Effect	Study	Source
G	0.0024	Lower sperm morphology.	Dasdag et al., 2015	emf-portal.org
H	0.0071	DNA damage in rat testes.	Akdag et al., 2016	researchgate.net
I	0.091	Oxidative stress in rat testes.	Atasoy et al., 2013	ncbi.nlm.nih.gov
J	0.4	DNA damage and lower motility in sperm.	De Luliis et al., 2009	journals.plos.org
K	1.2	Oxidative damage in testes.	Esmekaya et al., 2011	emf-portal.org
L	1.46	DNA damage and lower motility in sperm.	Zalata et al., 2015	emf-portal.org
M	2	Lower sperm morphology.	Falzone et al., 2011	ncbi.nlm.nih.gov

Annex 5

Chapter 5 — Can EMFs Affect Men's Fertility? (Meta-Analyses)

Year Of Publication	# Of Studies Looked At	Conclusion	Study	Source
2014	10	Mobile phone exposure negatively affects sperm quality.	Adams et al., 2014	sciencedirect.com
2012	26	Sperm exposed to RF radiation show decreased motility, morphometric abnormalities, and increased oxidative stress, whereas men using mobile phones have decreased sperm concentration, decreased motility and decreased viability.	La Vignera et al., 2012	ncbi.nlm.nih.gov
2009	99	RF from cell phones might affect the fertilizing potential of spermatozoa.	Desai et al., 2009	ncbi.nlm.nih.gov
2013	11	Mobile phone radiation has a tendency to significantly affect sperm quality.	Dama and Bhat, 2013	ncbi.nlm.nih.gov
2014	18	Evidence from current studies suggests potential harmful effects of mobile phone use on semen parameters.	Liu et al., 2014	ncbi.nlm.nih.gov
2016	27	RF is able to induce mitochondrial dysfunction [in sperm] leading to oxidative stress.	Houston et al., 2016	ncbi.nlm.nih.gov

Annex 6

Chapter 5 — Can EMFs Affect Your Head?

Table 1

Studies	RF Radiation (V/m)	Effect	Study	Source
A	0.14-0.39	Adults exposed to short-term cell phone radiation reported headaches, concentration difficulties (differences not significant, but elevated).	Thomas et al., 2008	ehjournal.biomedcentral.com
B	0.15	Impaired behavior in rats.	Daniels et al., 2009	emf-portal.org

Studies	RF Radiation (V/m)	Effect	Study	Source
C	0.24-0.89	Adults exposed to short-term GSM 900 radiation reported changes in mental state (e.g., calmness) but limitations of study on language descriptors prevented refined word choices (stupified, zoned-out).	Augner et al., 2009	ncbi.nlm.nih.gov
D	0.55	Impaired memory in ants.	Cammaerts et al., 2012	emf-portal.org
E	0.7	RFR from 3G cell towers decreased cognition, well-being.	Zwamborn et al., 2003	emf-portal.org
F	0.78	Impaired behavior in ants.	Cammaerts et al., 2013	emf-portal.org
G	0.89-2.19	Adolescents and adults exposed only 45 min to UMTS cell phone radiation reported increases In headaches.	Riddervold et al., 2008	emf-portal.org
H	1.74-6.14	RFR caused emotional behavior changes, free-radical damage by super-weak MWs.	Akoev et al., 2002	ncbi.nlm.nih.gov
I	1.94	RFR induced pathological leakage of the blood-brain barrier.	Persson et al., 1997	link.springer.com
J	2.37	RFR reduced memory function in rats.	Nittby et al., 2007	emf-portal.org
K	8.68	Reduced neurotransmitters.	Aboul Ezz et al., 2013	ncbi.nlm.nih.gov
L	11.07-12.85	Effects on the cornea.	Akar et al., 2013	ncbi.nlm.nih.gov
M	13-34	Oxidative stress in rats brains.	Dasdag et al., 2012	emf-portal.org
N	14.31	Oxidative stress in rats brains.	Esmekaya et al., 2016	emf-portal.org
O	15.14	Changes in blood serotonin levels.	Eris et al., 2015	emf-portal.org
P	62.6	Structural changes in the frontal cortex, brain stem and cerebellum and impair the oxidative stress and inflammatory cytokine system.	Eser et al., 2013	turkishneurosurgery.org.tr

Table 2

Studies	RF Radiation (SAR W/kg)	Effect	Study	Source
Q	0.00067	Impaired memory and learning, DNA damage in brain.	Deshmukh et al., 2013	emf-portal.org
R	0.0016 - 0.0044	Very low power 700 MHz CW affects excitability of hippocampus tissue, consistent with reported behavioral changes.	Tattersall et al., 2001	ncbi.nlm.nih.gov
S	0.016-2	Decreased neuron formation.	Bas et al., 2009	ncbi.nlm.nih.gov
T	0.17-0.58	Oxidative stress in rats brains.	Dasdag et al., 2009	emf-portal.org
U	0.31-0.78	DNA damage to bone marrow.	Sekeroglu and Sekeroglu, 2013	ncbi.nlm.nih.gov
V	0.37	Changes in brain metabolism in rats.	Fragopoulou et al., 2012	emf-portal.org
W	0.41-0.98	Impaired memory in rats.	Fragopoulou et al., 2010	emf-portal.org
X	1.38-1.45	Neurotoxic biomarkers in rats.	Carballo-Quintás et al., 2011	ncbi.nlm.nih.gov
Y	1.5	Stress in brain and nervous system.	Ammari et al., 2010	ncbi.nlm.nih.gov
Z	1.51	Long-term exposure to RF = microRNA expression changes in rats, links with neurodegenerative diseases.	Dasdag et al., 2015a	emf-portal.org
AA	1.6	DNA damage in human hair on the same side cell phone is used.	Cam and Seyhan, 2012	ncbi.nlm.nih.gov
BB	6h daily use of 3G phone for 10-40 days	Damage to nasal mucosa in rats, increased allergy symptoms.	Aydoğan et al., 2015	ncbi.nlm.nih.gov
CC	8h a day of exposure to a computer monitor	Oxidative stress in the eyes.	Mehmet et al., 2009	researchgate.net

Annex 7

Chapter 5 — Can EMFs Affect Your Weight?

Studies	RF Radiation (V/m)	Effect	Study	Source
A	0.04 - 0.9	Increase in salivary cortisol.	Augner et al., 2010	ncbi.nlm.nih.gov
B	0.15-0.19	Chronic exposure to base station RF (whole-body) in humans showed increased stress hormones; dopamine levels substantially decreased; higher levels of adrenaline and nor-adrenaline; dose-response seen; produced chronic physiological stress in cells even after 1.5 years.	Buchner and Eger, 2012	emf-portal.org
C	8.68	Increase in serum cortisol (a stress hormone).	Mann et al., 1998	emf-portal.org
D	43.41	A 24.6% drop in testosterone and 23.2% drop in insulin after 12 hrs of pulsed RFR exposure.	Navakatikian, 1994	In "*Biological Effects of Electric and Magnetic Fields, Volume 1*" D.O. Carpenter (ed) Academic Press, San Diego, CA, 1994, pp. 333-342. 1994

Annex 8

Chapter 5 — Can EMFs Affect Your Weight? (Exposure Type)

Type of Exposure	Effect	Study	Source
50-min cell phone call	50-minute cell phone exposure was associated with increased brain glucose metabolism in the region closest to the antenna.	Volkow et al., 2011	ncbi.nlm.nih.gov
One 30-min cell phone call per day for 80 days	Increase blood glucose levels in rats.	Celikozlu et al., 2012	ncbi.nlm.nih.gov
High levels of dirty electricity (>2,000 GS units)	Plasma glucose levels, in the Type 1 and Type 2 diabetic cases reported, respond to electromagnetic pollution in the form of radio frequencies in the kHz range associated with indoor wiring (dirty electricity).	Havas, 2008	ncbi.nlm.nih.gov

Type of Exposure	Effect	Study	Source
High levels of dirty electricity (>2,000 GS units)	Reduced blood sugar levels after Dirty Electricity filters were installed.	Sogabe, 2006	Sogabe, K. (2006). Yoyogi Natural Clinic in Japan. Personal communication, July 11.
Magnetic fields above 6 mG	Increased blood glucose levels.	Litovitz et al., 1994	Litovitz T. A., Eisenberg K. S., Tatlor T. *Effect of 60 Hz magnetic fields on blood glucose levels of diabetic humans and its inhibition by EM noise.* 16th Annu. Meeting Bioelectromagn. Soc.; June 12–17; Copenhagen, Denmark. 1994. p. 128.

Annex 9

Chapter 5 — Can EMFs Affect Your Heart? (RF)

Table 1

Studies	RF Radiation (V/m)	Effect	Study	Source
A	0.05-0.22	Cardio-vascular problems.	Oberfeld, 2004	vws.org
B	0.43-0.61	Adverse neurological, cardio symptoms and cancer risk.	Khurana et al., 2010	ncbi.nlm.nih.gov
C	1.19	Calcium metabolism in heart cells.	Schwartz et al., 1990	emf-portal.org
D	3.07	Calcium concentrations in heart muscle cells.	Wolke et al., 1996	onlinelibrary.wiley.com
E	20	Changes in blood pressure and heart rate.	Szmigielski et al., 1998	ncbi.nlm.nih.gov

Table 2

Studies	RF Radiation (SAR W/kg)	Effect	Study	Source
F	0.00015 - 0.003	Calcium ion movement in isolated frog heart tissue is increased 18% (P<.01) and by 21% (P<.05) by weak RF field modulated at 16 Hz.	Schwartz et al., 1990	ncbi.nlm.nih.gov
G	0.48	Changes in HRV.	Andrzejak et al., 2008	emf-portal.org
H	1	Changes in HRV.	Huber et al., 2003	emf-portal.org
I	1.2	Oxidative damage in heart.	Esmekaya et al., 2011	emf-portal.org

Annex 10

Chapter 5 — Can EMFs Affect Your Heart? (MF)

Studies	MF Radiation (mG)	Effect	Study	Source
A	0.00034	Altered heart rate in dogs.	Scherlag et al., 2004	ncbi.nlm.nih.gov
B	24	Decreased antioxidant levels in heart.	Martinez-Samano et al., 2010	emf-portal.org
C	42	Changes in HRV.	Baldi et al., 2007	emf-portal.org
D	373	Changes in HRV, blood pressure.	Bortkiewicz et al., 2006	emf-portal.org
E	800	Increased blood pressure, reduced HRV.	Ghione et al., 2004	onlinelibrary.wiley.com

Annex 11

Chapter 5 — Can EMFs Affect Your Detox?

Studies	RF Radiation (SAR W/kg)	Effect	Study	Source
A	0.14	Elevated levels of antibodies in spleen.	Elekes et al., 1996	emf-portal.org
B	0.38	Oxidative damage in liver.	Ozgur et al., 2010	ncbi.nlm.nih.gov

Studies	RF Radiation (SAR W/kg)	Effect	Study	Source
C	0.6	DNA damage in kidney and liver.	Trosic et al., 2011	emf-portal.org
D	0.88	Oxidative damage in liver.	Furtado-Filho et al., 2014	emf-portal.org
E	1.2	Oxidative damage in liver.	Esmekaya et al., 2011	emf-portal.org
F	1.2	Oxidative stress in kidneys.	Ozorak et al., 2013	ncbi.nlm.nih.gov
G	1.52	Oxidative stress on bladder tissue.	Koca et al., 2014	ncbi.nlm.nih.gov
H	1.6	Oxidative damage in liver cells.	Luo et al., 2014	ncbi.nlm.nih.gov

Annex 12

Chapter 5 — Can EMFs Affect Your Children? (RF)

Table 1

Studies	RF Radiation (V/m)	Effect	Study	Source
A	0.11-0.27	Short-term exposure in children and teens caused headache, irritation, concentration difficulties in school.	Heinrich et al., 2010	emf-portal.org
B	0.33-1.02	Increase in ADHD.	Calvente et al., 2016	ncbi.nlm.nih.gov
C	0.78	Motor function, memory and attention of school children affected.	Kolodynski and Kolodynska, 1996	ncbi.nlm.nih.gov
D	0.87-5.49	Two-fold increase in leukemia in children.	Hocking et al., 1996	emf-portal.org
E	0.87-5.49	Decreased survival in children with leukemia.	Hocking et al., 2000	emf-portal.org
F	2.17	Impaired kidney development in rats (in-utero exposure).	Pyrpasopoulou et al., 2004	ncbi.nlm.nih.gov
G	25-35	Impaired bone growth in mouse embryos.	Fragopoulou et al., 2010	emf-portal.org

Table 2

Studies	RF Radiation (SAR W/kg)	Effect	Study	Source
H	0.6-0.9	Impaired bone growth in mouse fetuses.	Fragopoulou et al., 2009	avaate.org
I	1.6	Mice fetuses exposed to RF developed ADHD symptoms as adults.	Aldad et al., 2012	nature.com
J	1.98	Changes in brain waves in children (consequences unclear).	Krause et al., 2006	emf-portal.org

Annex 13

Chapter 5 — Can EMFs Affect Your Children? (MF)

Studies	MF Radiation (mG)	Effect	Study	Source
K	2	Increased risk for leukemia in children exposed to fields of 2mG or higher.	Zhao et al., 2014	ncbi.nlm.nih.gov
L	2	Increased risk for leukemia in children exposed to fields of 2mG or higher.	Feychting and Ahlbom, 1993	emf-portal.org
M	4	Significant increased risk for 3 types of childhood cancers.	Olsen et al., 1993	emf-portal.org
N	10	60 Hz magnetic field could inhibit the development of the vascular system in quail embryos.	Costa and de Albuquerque, 2015	emf-portal.org
O	15	Prenatal exposure to magnetic field level (> 0.15 μT) was associated with increased risk of being obese in offspring compared with a lower magnetic field level below 0.15 μT (OR 1.7, CI 1.01-2.84).	Li et al., 2012	emf-portal.org
P	30	Prenatal and neonatal exposure to extremely low frequency magnetic fields could impair the infant rat myocardium.	Tayefi et al., 2010	emf-portal.org

Annex 14

Chapter 5 — Can EMFs Affect Your Children? (Other Studies)

Findings	Study	Source
Combined exposure to environmental lead and mobile phone increases risks of ADHD.	Byun et al., 2013	journals.plos.org
Associations between cell phone use and behavioral problems in young children.	Divan et al., 2012	emf-portal.org
Children's skulls absorb way more radiation than those of adults.	Gandhi, O. P., 2015	ieeexplore.ieee.org
10 year-old children absorb 153% more radiation than adults.	Gandhi, O. P. et al., 2012	tandfonline.com
Children 11-15 years old using cell phones suffer have an increased risk for headaches, migraines and skin itches.	Chiu et al., 2015	emf-portal.org
Cell phone use in teenagers increase behavioral problems.	Thomas et al., 2010	emf-portal.org
Cell phone use increases risks of brain tumors, even at low exposures.	Söderqvist et al., 2011	ehjournal.net
Positive relationship between cell phone use in children and increased risk for brain tumors.	Morgan et al., 2012	researchgate.net
The relationship between MF and childhood leukemia remains consistent with possible carcinogenicity in humans.	Schuz et al., 2016	ncbi.nlm.nih.gov
500% increase brain cancer risk for teenagers using cell phones before age 20.	Hardell and Carlberg, 2013	ncbi.nlm.nih.gov

Annex 15

Chapter 6 — RF Guidelines Around The World

Authority	Safety Limit (V/m)	Notes & References
USA (FCC)	61.4	—
Belgium	21	—
Russia, China	6	powerwatch.org.uk
EUROPAEM EMF Guidelines	0.02	At night, for a wifi router. researchgate.net
Building Biology (Slight Anomaly)	0.06	In sleep areas. createhealthyhomes.com

Authority	Safety Limit (V/m)	Notes & References
Bioinitiative Report, 2012	0.03	bioinitiative.org
Austria	0.02	—
Mother Nature	0.00002	As reported by Michael Bevington in Electromagnetic Sensitivity and Electromagnetic Hypersensitivity. es-uk.info

Annex 16

Chapter 6 — MF Guidelines Around The World

Authority	Safety Limit (mG)	Notes & References
International (IEEE)	9,040	For exposure to the head and torso.
International (ICNIRP)	2,000	emfs.info
Council of the European Union	1,000	—
Argentina	250	—
Brazil	30	Investigation levels for the city of Sao Paulo.
Switzerland	10	—
Netherlands, Norway	4	—
Israel	2	Chronic exposure, annual average.
Lowest level linked with childhood cancers	2	emfcenter.com
EUROPAEM EMF Guidelines	1	Nighttime exposure. researchgate.net
Building Biology (Slight Anomaly)	1	In sleeping areas. createhealthyhomes.com
Bioinitiative Report, 2012	1	bioinitiative.org
Mother Nature	0.000002	As reported by Michael Bevington in Electromagnetic Sensitivity and Electromagnetic Hypersensitivity. es-uk.info

Annex 17

Chapter 6 — EF Guidelines Around The World

Authority	Safety Limit (V/m)	Notes & References
International (IEEE)	10,000	Investigation level under normal load conditions.
International (ICNIRP)	5,000	—
Council of the European Union	5,000	—
Argentina	3,000	—
Costa Rica	2,000	At border of right of way.
Poland	1,000	Residential areas.
Russia, Slovenia	500	Residential buildings.
Building Biology (Slight Anomaly)	1.5	Field strength potential-free in sleep areas. createhealthyhomes.com
EUROPAEM EMF Guidelines	1	Nighttime exposure. researchgate.net
Mother Nature	0.0001	As reported by Michael Bevington in Electromagnetic Sensitivity and Electromagnetic Hypersensitivity. es-uk.info

PHOTO CREDITS

Photo Credits

Chapter 3

Nokia 9000 — Picture by Oldmobil — upload.wikimedia.org/wikipedia/commons/8/88/Nokia-9110-9000.jpg.
CC BY-SA 3.0 creativecommons.org/licenses/by-sa/3.0/deed.en

SAM's Head — Photo by Jaume Anguera. researchgate.net/profile/Jaume_Anguera2publication/255171502/figure/fig25/AS:324945109372988@1454484359950/A-model-of-the-specific-anthropomorphic-mannequin-SAM-head.png.
CC BY 3.0 creativecommons.org/licenses/by/2.0/

SAM Cell Phone Testing Equipment — screenshot from CBC's Marketplace exposé "The secret inside your cell phone". Retrieved on June 25th 2017. See youtube.com/watch?v=Wm69ik_Qdb8&app=desktop

Chapter 4

Ants Dance Around Smartphone — screenshot from YouTube ViralVideoLab's "Ants Circling My Phone - iphone ant control - Ameisen umkreisen iphone". Retrieved on June 25th 2017. See youtube.com/watch?v=GFX7mRl7xDs

VGCCs Pathways — Reproduced with minor aesthetic changes with the permission of Martin Pall, PhD. You can watch a more in-depth presentation of his work here: youtube.com/watch?v=Pjt0iJThPU0

Rat Brain With Compromised BBB — Photo by Mrs. Brigitte May. static-content.springer.com/esm/art%3A10.1186%2F2040-7378-4-6/MediaObjects/13231_2012_52_MOESM8_ESM.jpeg.
CC BY 2.0 creativecommons.org/licenses/by/2.0/

Chapter 5

Symptoms Experienced By People Near Cellular Phone Base Station — Based on the work of Santini et al., and used with the permission of Magda Havas, PhD. Used with the permission of Magda Havas, PhD.

iPotty — Photo by odels. flickr.com/photos/odels/8513383067/.
CC BY 2.0 creativecommons.org/licenses/by/2.0/

Chapter 6

Google Project Loon — Photo by ilitephoto. flickr.com/photos/ilitephoto/9052643301/in/photostream/.
CC BY 2.0 creativecommons.org/licenses/by/2.0/

Chapter 7

Eco-Wifi — Photo used with the permission of Dr. Jan-Rutger Schrader, PhD.

Hidden Cell Towers — From top to bottom. Picture #1 by SayCheeeeeese - upload.wikimedia.org/wikipedia/commons/b/b3/Cell_phone_tower_disguised_2008.jpg.
Picture #2 by Celltowerleases — upload.wikimedia.org/wikipedia/commons/c/c2/Flagpole_Monopole_Concealed_Cell_Tower.jpg.
Picture #3 by Pplecke — upload.wikimedia.org/wikipedia/commons/a/a0/BTS_NodeB_antenna_Sopot.jpg.
Picture #4 by Minnaert — upload.wikimedia.org/wikipedia/commons/6/66/PalmCellTower.jpg.
CC BY 2.0 creativecommons.org/licenses/by/2.0/

Fluorescent Light Under Power Lines — Picture by BaronAlaric - commons.wikimedia.org/wiki/File:Fluorescent_tube_under_electric_line.jpg#/media/File:Fluorescent_tube_under_power_lines_SETUP.JPG.
CC BY-SA 3.0 creativecommons.org/licenses/by-sa/3.0/

Printed in Great Britain
by Amazon